Cocaine: Physiological and Physiopathological Effects

The *Journal of Addictive Diseases* series:*
(formerly *Advances in Alcohol & Substance Abuse* series)

- *Behavioral and Biochemical Issues in Substance Abuse**
- *Cocaine, AIDS, and Intravenous Drug Use**
- *What Works in Drug Abuse Epidemiology**
- *Cocaine: Physiological and Physiopathological Effects**
- *Recent Advances in the Biology of Alcoholism*
- *The Effects of Maternal Alcohol and Drug Abuse on the Newborn*
- *Evaluation of Drug Treatment Programs*
- *Current Controversies in Alcoholism*
- *Federal Priorities in Funding Alcohol and Drug Abuse Programs*
- *Psychosocial Constructs of Alcoholism and Substance Abuse*
- *The Addictive Behaviors*
- *Conceptual Issues in Alcoholism and Substance Abuse*
- *Dual Addiction: Pharmacological Issues in the Treatment of Concomitant Alcoholism and Drug Abuse*
- *Cultural and Sociological Aspects of Alcholism and Substance Abuse*
- *Alcohol and Drug Abuse in the Affluent*
- *Alcohol and Substance Abuse in Adolescence*
- *Controversies in Alcoholism and Substance Abuse*
- *Alcohol and Substance Abuse in Women and Children*
- *Cocaine: Pharmacology, Addiction, and Therapy*
- *Children of Alcoholics*
- *Pharmacological Issues in Alcohol and Substance Abuse*
- *AIDS and Substance Abuse*
- *Alcohol Research from Bench to Bedside*
- *Addiction Potential of Abused Drugs and Drug Classes*

Cocaine: Physiological and Physiopathological Effects

Alfonso Paredes, MD
David A. Gorelick, MD, PhD
Guest Editors

Barry Stimmel, MD
Editor

The Haworth Press, Inc.
New York • London • Norwood (Australia)

Cocaine: Physiological and Physiopathological Effects has also been published as *Journal of Addictive Diseases,* Volume 11, Number 4, 1992.

The Haworth Press, Inc. 10 Alice Street, Binghamton, NY 13904-1580 USA

Library of Congress Cataloging-in-Publication Data

Cocaine : physiological and physiopathological effects / Alfonso Paredes, David A. Gorelick, guest editors; Barry Stimmel, editor .

p. cm.

"Has also been published as Journal of addictive diseases, volume 11, number 4, 1992"–T.p. verso.

Includes bibliographical references.

ISBN 1-56024-311-2 (acid-free paper).–ISBN 1-56024-385-6 (pbk.) (acid-free paper)

1. Cocaine–Physiological effect. 2. Cocaine–Pathophysiology. I. Paredes, Alfonso. II. Gorelick, David A. III. Stimmel, Barry, 1939- .

QP801.C68C65 1992

615'.785–dc20 92-19390

CIP

Cocaine: Physiological and Physiopathological Effects

CONTENTS

ABOUT THE GUEST EDITORS

Alfonso Paredes, MD, is a member of the staff of the Substance Abuse Programs at the West Los Angeles Veterans Affairs Medical Center (Brentwood Division) and Professor of Psychiatry and Biobehavioral Sciences at the School of Medicine, University of California, Los Angeles. Doctor Paredes has numerous publications covering topics on the behavioral effects of alcohol in humans and clinical and experimental research in alcohol and cocaine dependence.

David A. Gorelick, MD, PhD, is a medical graduate from the Albert Einstein College of Medicine, Bronx NY and received his PhD from the same institution. Dr. Gorelick is a former chief of the Behavioral Pharmacology Laboratory at the West Los Angeles Veterans Affairs Medical Center (Brentwood Division) and a member of the UCLA faculty. Presently he is Chief, Treatment and Early Intervention Branch, National Institute on Drug Abuse and Clinical Professor of Psychiatry at the University of Maryland School of Medicine. Dr. Gorelick is a neuroscientist and a clinical researcher with many publications covering basic and applied aspects in substance abuse.

∞ ALL HAWORTH BOOKS & JOURNALS
ARE PRINTED ON CERTIFIED
ACID-FREE PAPER

EDITORIAL

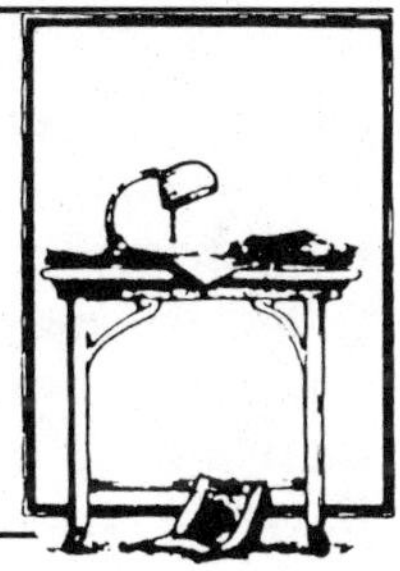

Physiological and Physiopathological Effects of Cocaine

A brief review of the extent to which illicit drugs are used in this country may place in perspective the role of cocaine as a public health hazard. According to the National Household Survey on Drug Abuse, 37% of the population older than 12 report having used drugs.[1] Fourteen percent have used within the past year and 7% the last month. In actual numbers the size of the user population is substantial. The rates quoted suggest that an estimated 72 million people have been exposed to illicit drugs during their lifetime and 14 million have consumed these agents within the past month.

There are significant differences in preference between the various drugs. Marijuana is the most popular with 33% of the surveyed population reporting having used it, second is cocaine with 10% mentioning use. Next in decreasing order are the hallucinogens followed by other stimulants such as amphetamines. It may be noted in passing that the drugs that may be purchased legally such as alcohol and tobacco, which in many circumstances are not less harmful, are considerably more popular with 85% and 78% of the surveyed population respectively reporting having consumed these substances.

The decade of the 1980's witnessed a remarkable increase in the self-reported prevalence of cocaine use. Population estimates from the National Institute on Drug abuse (NIDA) National Household Survey indicate that in 1990, 6.2 million Americans had used cocaine during the prior year, 662,000 used cocaine at least weekly, and 336,000 daily.[2]

The experience of clinicians, emergency rooms, and medical examiners as well as dramatic accounts in the mass media, indicate that the use of cocaine carries serious health risks. Cocaine associated hospital emergency room visits reported to NIDA's Drug Abuse Warning Network (DAWN) increased four-fold from 1985 to 1989, with 61,665 cocaine mentions in the last year.[3] Cocaine was involved in 40% of all visits, it is therefore the most frequently mentioned drug. Cocaine use occurred in both sexes (67.1% male, 32.2% female) and among all races (25.2% white, 57.9% Black, 8.7% Hispanic). Patients in the 20-39 age range accounted for 83.4% of all the cocaine associated visits.

The severity of the cocaine associated episodes handled in hospital emergency rooms is reflected in the data reported by medical examiners to DAWN. In 1989, 3,618 cocaine-associated deaths were reported, a four-fold increase from 1985.[3] Cocaine was the number one drug mentioned accounting for 50.5% of all drug associated deaths reported. Cocaine-associated deaths involved both sexes (79.1% male, 20.4% female) and all races (36.1% white, 45.9% Black, 16.8% Hispanic). Patients 20-39 years old accounted for 72.2% of all cocaine-associated deaths.

One reason for the increasing morbidity and mortality associated with cocaine may be a shift in the preferred route of administration. The previously favored route of administration, intranasal "snorting" has been supplanted to a great extent by crack smoking and "freebasing." In the 1989 DAWN emergency room sample, 34.4% of the cocaine users smoked cocaine and 19.8% used it intravenously.[3] These methods deliver the drug in greater amounts and more efficiently. The intravenous route of administration brings additional risks such as HIV infection, hepatitis, and endocarditis. Smoking the alkaloid form of cocaine facilitates access of the drug to the CNS and the cardiovascular system through respiratory pathways and the extensive alveolar surface of the lung. Exposure to larger doses of the drug may account for more frequent and serious medical complications and very likely accelerates the induction of the addictive syndrome.

Given the magnitude of the health problems caused by cocaine, it is prudent to review closely the pathophysiological effects of the drug on major organ systems and identify needed areas for further research. This publication is devoted to these purposes. This information may help to increase awareness and understanding on the nature of the health risks of cocaine and their significance from individual and public health perspectives. Emergency rooms and other medical services such as general medicine, cardiology and neurology care for many patients with cocaine related problems who may not be referred for drug abuse rehabilitation. Clinicians working in rehabilitation therefore may underestimate the frequency and seriousness of cocaine-related medical complications.

The first article in this volume is a review by Wilkins of aspects of lung physiology relevant to cocaine.[4] The lung is important not only for its respiratory functions, but also for a number of metabolic, neuroendocrine and immunological functions which could be affected in the cocaine user. In the following paper, Kowatch and his team have reviewed the electroencephalographic sleep patterns associated with cocaine withdrawal.[5] His research found a persistence of the EEG changes following cocaine withdrawal. These patterns are similar to those observed in major depression and suggest a heightened pressure for REM sleep. It was observed that the time course for neurophysiological disturbances persist at least 5 weeks after discontinuation of the drug. This type of information may help us gain a better understanding of the pathophysiology of relapse and cocaine withdrawal.

An article by Miller and his group discusses the neurological problems associated with cocaine use and some of the changes observed with neuroimaging techniques.[6] The nervous system is vulnerable to the toxic effects of the drug at almost every anatomical and functional level. Cases have been reported of anterior spinal artery and lateral medullary syndromes, transient ischemic attacks including ischemic stroke and subarachnoid hemorrhage.[7,8] Mody et al. have reported complications such as ischemic infarcts in the territory of the middle cerebral artery, fronto temporal, right middle cerebral and vertebrobasilar arteries.[7] Seizures associated with cocaine use are common. This makes cocaine a leading risk factor for this problem among otherwise healthy young adults.[9] Considering the severity of neurological complications it is interesting that no more attention has been given to this area.

The paper by Tashkin and his associates examines the impact of cocaine on the respiratory functions of the lung assisted by data derived from their research.[10] Respiratory symptoms such as cough, black sputum, hemoptysis, dyspnea and chest pain are often reported by patients. Cases of pneumothorax and pneumomediastinum or diffuse lung damage have been mentioned in the literature.[11,12,13] It is therefore important to assess the nature of the damage to the lungs and small airways.

Other studies at the cellular level in lung tissues will be necessary. For example until recently the investigation of the macrophage function in the alveoli focused on the capacity to eliminate infectious agents. It is now apparent that these cells have important immunological functions such as secretion of interlukin-1 as well as the ability to act as accessory cells for lymphocytic proliferation. It remains to be determined if cocaine smoking acting on these mechanisms compromise the resistance to pathogens or increase the risk of lung neoplasia.[13]

The effects of cocaine on the cardiovascular system have been the source of considerable concern.[14,15,16] This area is reviewed by Nademanee.[17] He and his associates have conducted a series of interesting studies of cardiovascular function in cocaine users including 24-hour ambulatory Holter monitoring.[14] His work notes the importance of myocardial infarction in young cocaine users who otherwise, given their age would not be candidates for myocardial infarction. The normal coronary arteries found during postmortem examination and the presence of thrombi in their infarcted vessels, otherwise free of atherosclerotic plaques, implicate cocaine and the associated vasospasm as the factors responsible for infarction.

Other cardiovascular manifestations often observed in cocaine users include ventricular tachycardia, fibrillation, myocarditis and sudden death.[15,16,18] The seriousness of the cardiovascular responses is dramatized by reports of cases of aortic dissection.[19] Cardiovascular complications have physiological explanations. It has been shown that cocaine decreases blood flow of the coronary sinus and increases vascular resistance in segments such as the left coronary artery. The seriousness of these alterations is compounded by the increased myocardial oxygen demand.[20,21] It also has been suggested that coagulation functions are affected contributing to cocaine-induced thromboses.[21,22]

Other pathophysiological effects of cocaine not addressed in this issue deserve mention. Cases have been reported of hepatotoxicity,[23] hepatonecrosis[24] and acute renal failure.[25] Rhabdomyolisis[26,27] a relatively uncommon complication may deserve closer scrutiny. We have therefore included a paper by Warrian and associates reporting increased levels of creatinine phosphokinase in the urine of cocaine addicts.[28] This suggests toxic effects of the drug in the muscular system. General systemic reactions such as hyperthermia accompanied by status epilepticus and hypotension[29] constitute other serious complications. There is also some evidence that cocaine can directly affect the immune system.[30]

Of particular interest is the fact that pregnant women and the foetus are vulnerable. Women cocaine users show high rates of spontaneous abortion and abruptio placenta.[31,32] The neuropsychological functions of the newborn are also affected. For example, infants born to cocaine abusing mothers show significant deficits in interactive behavior and poor organizational responses to environmental stimuli. There is also evidence of low birth weight, intrauterine growth retardation and motor impairment.[33] A phenomenon mentioned in the literature is a decrease of cardiac output in infants of mothers who abuse cocaine.[34]

The closing paper by Gorelick provides a broad overview of the pathophysiology of cocaine, reviews some of the scientific issues relevant to the topic, and makes some suggestions for further research.[35]

The material presented in this issue reminds us that physicians and other health care workers, whether they focus their efforts primarily on the treatment of the addictive behavior or on the management of medical problems, need to become increasingly aware of the nature of the health consequences of cocaine use.

Alfonso Paredes
David A. Gorelick

REFERENCES

1. U.S. Department of Health and Human Services *National Household Survey on Drug Abuse: Population Estimates, 1988* DHHS Publication No. (ADM) 89-1636.

2. National Institute on Drug Abuse. *NIDA Notes* 1991; 5(5): 11-14.

3. U.S. Department of Health and Human Services *Data from the Drug Abuse Warning Network (DAWN) Annual Data 1989.* Series 1, Number 9 DHHS Publication No. (ADM) 90-1717, 1990.

4. Wilkins, J.N. Brain, lung, and cardiovascular interactions with cocaine and cocaine-induced catecholamine effects. *J. of Addictive Diseases* (1992) 11(4): 9-19.

5. Kowatch, R.A., Schnoll, S.S., Knisely, J.S. et al. Electroencephalographic sleep and mood during cocaine withdrawal. *J. of Addictive Diseases* (1992) 11(4): 21-45.

6. Miller, B.L., Mena, I., Giombetti, R. et al. Neuropsychiatric effects of cocaine: SPECT measurements. *J. of Addictive Diseases* (1992) 11(4): 47-58.

7. Mody, C.K., Miller, B.L., Mc Intyre et al. Neurologic complications of cocaine abuse *Neurology* 1988; 38: 1189-1193.

8. Nolte, K.B., Gelman, B.B. Intracerebral hemorrhage associated with cocaine abuse *Archives of Pathology and Laboratory Medicine* 1989; 113: 812-813.

9. Rowbotam, M.C., Lowenstein, D.H. Neurologic consequences of cocaine use. *Ann. Rev. Med.* 1990; 41: 417-422. N.J.

10. Tashkin, D.P., Gorelick, D., Khalsa, M., Simmons, M., Chang, P. Respiratory Effects of Cocaine Freebasing Among Habitual Cocaine Users. *J. of Addictive Diseases* (1992) 11(4): 59-70.

11. Morris, J.B., Schuck, J.M. Pneumomediastinum in a young male cocaine user. *Ann. Emerg. Med.* 1985; 14:194-196.

12. Schesser, R., Davis C., Edelstein S. Pneumomediastinum and pneumothorax after inhaling alkaloidal cocaine. *Ann. Emerg. Med.* 1981: 10:213-215.

13. Tashkin, D.P., Simmons, M.S., Coulson, A.H., Clark, V.A. and Goung Jr., H. Respiratory effects of cocaine "free basing" among habitual users of marijuana with or without tobacco *Chest* 1987; 92: 638-644.

14. Nademanee, K., Gorelick, D.A. et al. Myocardial ischemia during cocaine withdrawal *Ann. Intern. Med* 1989; 876-880.

15. Cregler, L.L., Mark, H. Cardiovascular dangers of cocaine abuse *Am. J. Cardiol.* 1986; 57: 1185-1186.

16. Isner, J.M., Estes, N.A. Thompson et al. Acute cardiac events temporarily related to cocaine abuse. *New Engl. J. of Med.* 1986; 315:1438-1443.

17. Nademanee, K. Cardiovascular Effects and Toxicities of Cocaine. *J. of Addictive Diseases* (1992) 11(4): 71-82.

18. Lathers, C.C., Spino, M.M. et al. Cocaine induced seizures, arrhythmia and sudden death. In C.M. Lathers and P.L. Schroeder (eds.) *Epilepsy and Sudden Death.* New York; Dreker 1991 pp 343-415.

19. Gadaleta, D., Hall, M.N, Cocaine induced aortic dissection *Chest* 1989; 96: 1203-1205.

20. Lange, R.A., Cigarroa, R.C., Yancy C.W. et al. Cocaine induced coronary artery vasoconstriction *New Engl. J. Med.* 1989; 321: 1557-1562.

21. Isner, J.M., Chokshi, S.K. Cocaine and vasospasm *New Engl. J. Med.* 1989; 321:1604-1606.

22. Chokshi S.K., Miller G., Rongione, A. Isner, J.M. Cocaine and cardiovascular diseases: The leading edge. *Cardiology* III 1989; 1-6.

23. Wanless, I.R., Dore, S., Gopinath N. et al. Histopathology of cocaine hepatotoxicity: Report of four patients *Gastroenterology* 1990; 98: 497-501.

24. Perino, L.E.,Warren, G.H.., Levine, J.S. Cocaine induced hepatotoxicity in humans *Gastroenterology* 1987; 93:176-180.

25. Singhal, P., Horowitz, B. Quinones, M.C. et al. Acute renal failure following cocaine abuse *Nephron* 1989; 52: 76-78.

26. Herzlich, B.C., Arsura E.L., Pagala, M., Grob D. Rhabdomyolysis related to cocaine abuse *Ann. Intern. Med.* 1988; 109:335-336.

27. Parks, J.M., Reed, G., Knochel, J.P. Cocaine associated rhabdomyolysis *American Journal of Medical Sciences* 1989; 297: 334-336.

28. Warrian, W.G., Halikas, J.A., Crosby, R.D. et al. Observations on increased CPK levels in "asymptomatic" cocaine abusers. *J. of Addictive Diseases* (1992) 11(4):83-85.

29. Campbell, B.G. Cocaine abuse and hyperthermia, seizures and fatal complications *Medical J. of Australia* 1988; 149: 387-389.

30. Ou, D.W., Shen, M.L., Luo, Y.P. Effects of cocaine and the immune system of Balb/C mice *Clin. Immunopathol.* 1989; 52: 305-312.

31. Little, B.B., Snell, L.M., Klein, V., Gilstrap L.C. III Cocaine abuse during pregnancy: maternal and fetal implications *Obstetrics and Gynecology* 1989; 73: 157-160.

32. Wang C.H. Schnoll, S.H. Prenatal cocaine use associated with down regulation of receptors in human placenta *Neurotoxicology and Teratology* 1987; 9: 301-304.

33. Chesnoff, I.J., Griffith, D.R., Mac Gregor et al. Temporal pattern of cocaine use in pregnancy: perinatal outcome *J.A.M.A.* 1989; 261: 1741-1744.

34. Van de Bor, M., Walther, F.J. Ephraimi, M. Decreased cardiac output in infants of mothers who abused cocaine. *Pediatrics* 1990; 85: 30-32.

35. Gorelick, D.A. Pathophysiological Effects of Cocaine in Humans: Review of Scientific Issues. *J. of Addictive Diseases* (1992) 11(4):97-100.

Brain, Lung, and Cardiovascular Interactions with Cocaine and Cocaine-Induced Catecholamine Effects

Jeffery N. Wilkins, MD

SUMMARY. The pathophysiologic effects of cocaine on neuronal, pulmonary, and cardiovascular tissue are related to the drug's interaction with select catecholamine and neuroendocrine systems. Cocaine has been shown to alter circulating levels of the neurotransmitters, dopamine, norepinephrine, epinephrine, as well as the hypothalamic-pituitary-adrenal axis hormones corticotropin-releasing factor (CRF), adrenocorticotropic hormone (ACTH), and cortisol. Furthermore, brain and lung tissue have been identified as primary sites of cocaine sequestration and metabolism. This paper reviews evidence suggesting that steroid-potentiated actions of catecholamines on vascular tissues contributes to the etiology of cocaine-related medical complications, including ischemic stroke, coronary ischemia, and ischemia-based renal failure.

INTRODUCTION

This paper examines brain uptake of cocaine, cocaine-induced increases in select catecholamines and hormones, and the role these catecholamines and hormones may play in cocaine-related medical complications. First, the mechanisms by which the brain removes

---

Jeffery N. Wilkins is Chief, Substance Abuse Programs, West Los Angeles VAMC, Brentwood Division, 11301 Wilshire Blvd., Los Angeles, CA 90073 and Associate Adjunct Professor of Psychiatry, UCLA School of Medicine.

The author wishes to express his appreciation to David Herzberg for his creative and editorial assistance in the preparation of this manuscript.

cocaine from blood and the role of the lung as a site of cocaine sequestration are discussed. Second, the paper describes the effect of cocaine on circulating levels of select catecholamines, including dopamine (DA), epinephrine (E), and norepinephrine (NE), as well as on corticotropin-releasing factor (CRF), adrenocorticotropic hormone (ACTH), and cortisol. Third, the potential pathophysiologic impact of cocaine-released catecholamines on the brain, heart, and lung is examined. This latter discussion addresses some of the material presented by Drs. Miller, Nademanee, and Tashkin in this volume.

Discussion focuses on four hypotheses. These hypotheses, some of which are stated or implied in the writings of others (including other authors in this volume), are presented in the hope that further research will be conducted to evaluate their merits. The hypotheses are as follows:

1. Cocaine taken in large amounts (i.e., from inhalation of crack or intravenous administration) is initially sequestered by the lung. Some of the cocaine is metabolized, but the bulk is subsequently released over time into the blood stream for uptake into other tissues including the brain.
2. Cocaine reliably produces increases in circulating levels of norepinephrine, epinephrine, and dopamine as well as corticosteroids.
3. Steroid-potentiated actions of catecholamines on vascular tissues contributes to the etiology of cocaine-related medical complications including ischemic stroke, coronary ischemia, and ischemia-based renal failure.
4. Catecholamine depletion resulting from chronic cocaine use may alter airway resistance dynamics, and thus potentially exacerbate asthma.

BRAIN AND LUNG UPTAKE OF COCAINE

The ability of a drug to permeate the blood-brain barrier is related to the drug molecule's relative affinity for the four types of molecules present at the barrier: plasma water, plasma proteins, membrane lipid, and membrane carrier proteins. Although the absolute solubility in lipids is relevant, the most important factor governing a drug's permeability is its relative affinity for lipids verses its affinity for water.[1] In rat brain, cocaine has been shown to have a brain uptake index[1a] of 99.5 ± 3.4 S.D.[2] The high ratio indicates that the drug has an almost 100 fold potential to be taken up in the lipid, and thus crosses the blood-brain barrier with relative ease.

The brain also has been shown to be a site of sequestration of peripheral metabolites of cocaine. Benuck et al.[3] gave intraperitoneal injections of cocaine to mice and recorded brain and plasma levels of norcocaine (NC) and N-hydroxynorcocaine (NHNC), two oxidative metabolites of cocaine. Changes in brain NHNC levels were found to mirror changes in plasma NHNC concentrations. Since no appreciable amounts of NC or NHNC were measured in the brain following intracisternal administration of cocaine to mice, the authors of this study concluded that most of metabolites found in brain result from plasma metabolic processes, rather than from cerebral oxidative metabolism.

When first administered, many psychopharmacologic agents are sequestered by the lung to a greater degree than by other tissues. As with brain uptake, pulmonary uptake is dependent on the relative lipophilicity of the drug. Unlike brain uptake, the degree of uptake into the lung also depends on the drug's pKa. In seminal work in this area, Orton et al.,[4] Anderson et al.,[5] and Eling et al.[6] examined the removal mechanisms of numerous drugs, including psychopharmacologic amines, in perfused lungs. Their data indicate that amine containing drugs must have a pKa greater than eight and substantial lipophilic character to facilitate efficient uptake from the pulmonary circulation. Psychopharmacologic amines with these characteristics include chlorpromazine, desipramine, diphenhydramine, fluphenazine, imipramine, methadone, promazine, and propranolol. We have presented data demonstrating that phencyclidine (PCP) also follows this pattern.[7] According to the Orton, Anderson, and Eling

---

[1a] Brain Uptake Index (BUI) = $[(\text{brain}\,^{14}C/\text{brain}\,^{3}H)/(\text{injected}\,^{14}C/\text{injected}\,^{3}H)] - [(\text{brain}\,^{113m}In/\text{brain}\,^{3}H)/(\text{injected}\,^{113m}In/\text{injected}\,^{3}H)] \times 100$

studies, the mechanism for uptake of these psychopharmacologic amines consists of facilitated diffusion driven by intracellular binding of the amines. However, unique, highly specific transport mechanisms can also exist, as demonstrated by Philpot et al.[8] These investigators found that lung uptake of amphetamine takes place through a carrier-mediated mechanism, presumably the same carrier that transports NE, in light of the structural similarities between amphetamine and NE.

Our first hypothesis is that when cocaine is administered it is distributed to all tissues by the blood but with the lung as the predominate initial site for tissue sequestration. This follows from cocaine's demonstrated lipophilicity, its pKa[9] of 8.5, and its chemical similarity to compounds that do accumulate in the lung. Although cocaine held in the lung is subject to metabolism (most of the enzymes required for biotransformation of psychopharmacologic compounds are found in the lung[10,11]), it is doubtful that significant metabolism of intravenous or smoked "crack" cocaine occurs in the lung. Due to the significant levels of cocaine absorbed into the blood stream from these modes of administration, much of the drug would likely be released back into the bloodstream without undergoing metabolism. This unmetabolized cocaine would then be available for uptake by other viscera.

CATECHOLAMINE AND STEROID RESPONSES TO COCAINE

Many of cocaine's acute actions in the brain and in other tissues, and possibly its chronic actions as well, appear to be secondary to its ability to release endogenous substrates, including select catecholamines and steroids. Our second hypothesis proposes that cocaine reliably produces increases in circulating levels of norepinephrine, epinephrine, and dopamine as well as corticosteroids. Catecholamine levels rise with acute cocaine administration (see discussion below), while chronic administration is assumed to produce decreased catecholamine levels, and may also potentiate catecholamine receptor sensitivity. For example, it has been hypothesized that chronic dopamine depletion may explain the dysphoric aspects of cocaine withdrawal.[12]

In a preliminary study, cocaine infusion has been shown to acutely increase circulating levels of dopamine, norepinephrine, and epinephrine in cocaine-dependent humans.[13] These findings have been supported in studies in the dog and squirrel monkey. Schwartz et al.[14] measured plasma catecholamine levels in conscious dogs infused with cocaine at a rate of 2.8 ± 1.2 mg/kg. Plasma DA, NE, and E concentrations in the experimental group were two to three times higher than those of the control group. Furthermore, plasma catecholamine levels remained elevated throughout the study even though plasma cocaine levels decreased. In a study of the effects of nimodipine on cocaine-induced physiological alterations in the squirrel monkey, Trouve et al.[15] measured significant increases in plasma concentrations of DA, NE, and E following 0.5, 1, and 2 mg/kg intravenous cocaine injections.

The hypothalamic-pituitary-adrenal axis (HPA) has also been demonstrated to be stimulated by acute cocaine administration. For example, single cocaine infusions produced dose-dependent increases in ACTH levels, while repeated injections did not increase peripheral levels of ACTH.[16] The mechanism of this stimulation is as yet unclear. For example, Moldow and Fischman[17] observed significant increases in plasma ACTH, ß-endorphin, and corticosterone concentrations in rats following cocaine administration. However, injection of cocaine did not produce a significant change in hypothalamic corticotropin releasing factor like immunoreactivity (CRF-LI) concentrations compared to saline-injected controls. In addition, rats pretreated with a preparation that blocks the release of endogenous CRF showed increased corticosterone concentrations after cocaine injection. These findings suggest that the anterior pituitary gland mediates the release of ACTH and ß-endorphin following cocaine administration. In contrast, Rivier and Vale[18] found that cocaine-induced elevation of rat ACTH levels was aborted by pretreatment with a CRF antiserum These results suggest that cocaine can act on the pituitary only in the presence of endogenous CRF, suggesting that the drug stimulates the release of endogenous CRF. Measurements of cocaine-induced steroid alterations in humans appear limited to studies of cocaine withdrawal. Mendelson et al.[19] investigated cortisol and testosterone levels in male cocaine abusers undergoing withdrawal, but found no significant alterations in the circulating levels of these hormones.

In humans, prolactin (HPrl) has been reported to be elevated following cocaine withdrawal.[19, 20] Rats receiving multiple 1 mg/kg infusions of cocaine over a period of ten days manifested incremental increases of pre-infusion HPrl concentrations in a time-dependent manner. This contrasts with the decreases found in post-infusion HPrl levels.[16] Interestingly, in this same study single infusions of cocaine in male rats did not significantly alter plasma prolactin concentrations. These results suggest that the repeated cocaine dosing schedule produced altered hypothalamic dopaminergic activity, since dopamine is known to regulate HPrl secretion.[21]

TISSUE INTERACTIONS WITH COCAINE-INDUCED CATECHOLAMINES

As described in other chapters of this volume, cocaine is associated with a number of medical complications, including stroke, coronary ischemia, and renal failure. We hypothesize that many of these medical disorders associated with acute and chronic cocaine self-administration may be due to the steroid-potentiated actions of cocaine-enhanced catecholamines on the vascular tissues of the brain, heart, and kidney, respectively. Several studies have shown that the presence of certain steroids can affect the interaction between circulating catecholamines and specific tissues. In particular, Iversen and Salt[22] demonstrated that various steroids (17-ß-oestradiol, corticosterone, deoxycorticosterone, progesterone, testosterone, and androsterone) produce a dose-dependent inhibition of the uptake of NE in the isolated rat heart. The uptake, and hence subsequent metabolism, of both unchanged NE and its metabolites was inhibited by the steroids, indicating that the steroids acted primarily on uptake rather than on metabolic mechanisms.

Considerable evidence supports a relationship between ischemic stroke and changes in brain catecholamines. For example, Minegishi et al.[23] found significant elevations in plasma catecholamines in patients with subarachnoid hemorrhage. In a study of 21 patients with acute brain infarction, Wester et al.[24] measured CSF levels of monoamine metabolites. Elevated concentrations of 3-methoxytyramine, homovanillic acid (a dopamine metabolite), 5-hydroxyindoleacetic acid (a serotonin metabolite) were observed. Gandhavadi[25] reported a case of a patient with brainstem stroke experiencing paroxysms of hypertension. Serum concentrations of DA, NE, and E were elevated during the episode, returning to normal after the paroxysms subsided. In a study of ten elderly stroke patients, Jansen et al.[26] observed a significant correlation between blood pressure after stroke and urinary E and NE. The results indicate that post-stroke modulation of blood pressure is mediated in part by changes in catecholamine production.

The human stroke data is supported by the results of animal studies. For example, Smith et al.[27] investigated the effect of permanent obstruction of the left middle cerebral artery on plasma catecholamine levels in cats. Significant elevations of plasma NE (33%), E (44%), and DA (28%) were observed. Similarly, Solomon et al.[28] observed a 64% increase in tissue concentration of NE in the brains of rats, 72 hours after experimental subarachnoid hemorrhage.

In addition to the acute respiratory tract injury caused by "crack" cocaine smoking (e.g., Tashkin et al., this volume), lung abnormalities, including asthma, may be affected by the altered plasma catecholamine concentrations associated with cocaine use. Our fourth hypothesis suggests that depletion of catecholamines by chronic cocaine use may alter airway resistance dynamics and thus potentially exacerbate asthma. The literature has established that altered plasma levels of certain catecholamines affect the symptoms of bronchial asthma. Subcutaneous injection of epinephrine is a well-known treatment for severe asthma attacks.[29-31] In addition, decreased epinephrine secretion is implicated in the bronchial obstruction found in nocturnal asthma.[32] In a study of asthmatic 3-to 11-year-olds and adolescents, Scanlon and Chang[33] observed decreased levels of NE and increased levels of its metabolite, MHPG. The authors interpreted these results as suggesting that brain NE plays an important role in the beta-adrenergic dysfunction characteristic of bronchial asthma. In a study of exercise-induced asthma, Pichurko et al.[34] found that plasma levels of NE rose with bronchodilation and fell with bronchoconstriction. These investigators also observed that exogenously administered NE consistently abolished the bronchial narrowing produced by exercise. Zimmerman and Nagel[35] found that children suffering from nocturnal asthma have increased epinephrine and decreased DA levels.

CONCLUSION

A substantial amount of cocaine transfers through the lungs and into the blood stream from the smoking of "crack." This rate of absorption is supported by a massive bed of lung capillaries that prevent cocaine from entering the metabolic pathways of the GI-hepatic system. As the free base, cocaine is not charged and thus does not attract water through hydrogen bonding. Therefore, as a lipophilic drug, it is readily taken up through the blood-brain barrier into the brain, where it has powerful reinforcing properties.

Much of cocaine's dependency-producing capabilities appear to be secondary to its effects on the catecholamine systems, especially the dopamine-based reinforcement systems of the brain.[36] However, most of the drug remains in the periphery where it acts on a number of organ systems other than the brain. Upon administration, cocaine is readily taken up by the lung. Some metabolism may occur in the lung, but most of the drug is re-released back into the circulation over a time period of minutes Cocaine has a potent effect on circulating levels of catecholamines, especially in the first 10 minutes after administration. In addition, altered catecholamine levels can have profound effects on the functioning of the heart and other organs. Also, it has been demonstrated that corticosteroids, which may be also released by acute cocaine administration, potentiate the effects of catecholamines on vascular tissue. This steroid-potentiated catecholamine/vascular interaction may contribute to the pathophysiological basis for ischemic stroke, coronary ischemia, and renal dysfunction. Catecholamine depletion from chronic cocaine use may also play a role in exacerbations of asthma.

REFERENCES

1. Oldendorf, W. Certain aspects of drug distribution to brain. In: Levi G et al., ed. Transport Phenomena in the Nervous System. New York: Plenum Publishing, 1976.

2. Oldendorf, W. Clearance of radiolabeled substances by brain after arterial injection using a diffusible internal standard. In: Marks N, Rodnight R, ed. Research Methods in Neurochemistry, Vol. 5. New York: Plenum Publishing, 1981.

3. Orton TC, Anderson MW, Pickett RD, Eling TE, Fouts JE. Xenobiotic accumulation and metabolism by isolated perfused rabbit lungs. J Pharmacol Exp Ther. 1973; 186:482-97.

4. Benuck M, Reith M, Sershen H, Wiener H, Lajtha A. Oxidative metabolism of cocaine: comparison of brain and liver. Society for Experimental Biology and Medicine. 1989; 190:7-13.

5. Anderson MW, Orton TC, Pickett RD, Eling TE. Accumulation of amines in the isolated perfused rabbit lung. J Pharmacol Exp Ther. 1974; 189:456-66.

6. Eling TE, Pickett RD, Orton TC, Anderson MW. A study of the dynamics of imipramine accumulation in the isolated perfused rabbit lung. Drug Metab Disp. 1975; 3:389-400.

7. Wilkins JN, Majdecki J, Braun L, Oldendorf WH. Preferential binding of parenteral phencyclidine (PCP) by lung: comparison with brain, liver, fat, and plasma. Published in the Abstracts of the Proceedings of the CINP Congress, Clinical Neuropharmacology, Puerto Rico, 1986.

8. Philpot RM, Anderson MW, Eling TE. Uptake, accumulation, and metabolism of chemicals by the lung. In: Bakhle and Vane, ed. Metabolic Functions of the Lung. New York: Dekker; 1977

9. Merck Index, 11th Edition, S. Budavari ed. Merck and Co, 1989:2451.

10. Minchin RF, Boyd MR. Localization of metabolic activation and deactivation systems in the lung: significance to the pulmonary toxicity of xenobiotics. Ann Rev Pharmacol Toxicol. 1983; 23:217-38.

11. Bend JR, Serabjit-Singh CJ. Xenobiotic metabolism by extrahepatic tissues: relationship to target organ and cell toxicity. In: Mitchell JR, Horning MG ed. Drug Metabolism and Drug Toxicity. New York: Raven, 1984:99-136.

12. Dackis CA, Gold MS. New concepts in cocaine addiction: the dopamine depletion hypothesis. Neuroscience and Biobehavioral Reviews. 1985; 9(3):469-77.

13. Nademanee K, Gorelick DA, Josephson MA, Ryan MA, Wilkins JN, Robertson HA, Vaghaiwalle Mody F, Intarachot V. Myocardial ischemia during cocaine withdrawal. Annals of Internal Medicine. 1989; 111: 875-80.

14. Schwartz A, Boyle W, Janzen D, Jones R. Acute effects of cocaine on catecholamines and cardiac electrophysiology in the conscious dog. Canadian Journal of Cardiology. 1988; 4(4): 188-92.

15. Trouve R, Nahas GC, Manger WM, Vinyard C, Goldberg S. Interactions of nimodipine and cocaine on endogenous catecholamines in the squirrel monkey. Proceedings of the Society for Experimental Biology and Medicine. 1990; 193(3): 171-5.

16. Pilotte NS, Sharpe LG, Dax EM. Multiple, but not acute, infusions of cocaine alter the release of prolactin in male rats. Brain Research. 1990; 512(1): 107-12.

17. Moldow RL, Fischman AJ. Cocaine induced secretion of ACTH, beta-endorphin, and corticosterone. Peptides. 1987; 8(5):819-22.

18. Rivier C, Vale W. Cocaine stimulates adrenocorticotropin (ACTH) secretion through a corticotropin-releasing factor (CRF)-mediated mechanism. Brain Research. 1987; 422(2):403-6.

19. Mendelson JH, Teoh SK, Lange U, Mello NK, Weiss R, Skupny A, Ellingboe J. Anterior pituitary, adrenal, and gonadal hormones during cocaine withdrawal. American Journal of Psychiatry. 1988; 145(9): 1094-8.

20. Wilkins JN, Gorelick DA, Bamshad BR, Setoda DY. Elevated serum prolactin levels in newly abstinent male cocaine abusers. Abstract presented at Society for Neuroscience, Toronto, Canada, November, 1988.

21. MacLeod RM. Regulation of prolactin secretion. In: Martini L, Ganong WF ed. Frontiers In Neuroendocrinology. New York: Raven Press, 1976:169-194.

22. Iversen LL, Salt PJ. Inhibition of catecholamine Uptake$_2$ by steroids in the isolated rat heart. British Journal of Pharmacology. 1970; 40(3):528-30.

23. Minegishi A, Ishizaki T, Yoshida Y, Ahagon A, Shibata N, Kobayashi H. Plasma monoaminergic metabolites and catecholamines in subarachnoid hemorrhage. Clinical implications. Archives of Neurology. 1987; 44(4):423-8.

24. Wester P, Puu G, Reiz S, Winblad B, Wester PO. Increased monoamine metabolite concentrations and cholinesterase activities in cerebrospinal fluid of patients with acute stroke. Acta Neurologica Scandinavica. 1987; 76(6):473-9.

25. Gandhavadi B. Hypertension after brainstem stroke. Archives of Physical Medicine and Rehabilitation. 1988; 69(2):130-1.

26. Jansen PA, Thien T, Gribnau FW, Schulte BP, Willemsen JJ, Lamers KJ, Poels EF. Blood pressure and both venous and urinary catecholamines after cerebral infarction. Clinical Neurology and Neurosurgery. 1988; 90(1):41-5.

27. Smith KE, Hachinski VC, Gibson CJ, Ciriello J. Changes in plasma catecholamine levels after insula damage in experimental stroke. Brain Research. 1986; 375(1): 182-5.

28. Solomon RA, McCormack BM, Lovitz RN, Swift DM, Hegemann MT. Elevation of brain norepinephrine concentration after experimental subarachnoid hemorrhage. Neurosurgery. 1986; 19(3):363-6.

29. Cydulka R, Davison R, Grammer L, Parker M, Mathews J 4th. The use of epinephrine in the treatment of older adult asthmatics. Annals of Emergency Medicine. 1988; 17(4):322-6.

30. Naspitz CK, Sole D, Wandalsen N. Treatment of acute attacks of bronchial asthma. A comparative study of epinephrine (subcutaneous) and fenoterol (inhalation). Annals of Allergy. 1987; 59(1):21-4.

31. Lissac J, Labrousse J, Tenaillon A, Coulaud JM, Massart JD, Icole B. Treatment of severe acute asthma in adults. Annales de Medecine Interne. 1986; 137(1):34-7.

32. Busse WW. Pathogenesis and pathophysiology of nocturnal asthma. American Journal of Medicine. 1988; 85(1B):24-9.

33. Scanlon RT, Chang S. Brain norepinephrine: a possible role in bronchial asthma. Annals of Allergy. 1988; 60(4):333-8.

34. Pichurko BM, Sullivan B, Porcelli RJ, McFadden ER Jr. Endogenous adrenergic modification of exercise-induced asthma. Journal of Allergy and Clinical Immunology. 1986; 77(6):796-801.

35. Zimmermann T, Nagel M. Nocturnal changes in cortisol, catecholamines, cAMP and histamine in children with nocturnal bronchial asthma and in healthy children. Language: German. Klinische Padiatrie. 1987; 199(2): 103-7.

36. Kleber HD, Gawin FH. Cocaine abuse: a review of current and experimental treatments. NIDA Research Monograph Series, Vol 50, Cocaine: Pharmacology, Effects, and Treatment of Abuse, 1984.

Electroencephalographic Sleep and Mood During Cocaine Withdrawal

Robert A. Kowatch, MD
Sidney S. Schnoll, MD, PhD
Janet S. Knisely, PhD
Diane Green
Ronald K. Elswick, PhD

Robert A. Kowatch is affiliated with the Department of Psychiatry, University of Texas Southwestern Medical Center at Dallas, Dallas, TX. Sidney S. Schnoll is affiliated with the Department of Internal Medicine and the Department of Psychiatry, Division of Substance Abuse Medicine, Medical College of Virginia, Richmond, VA. Janet S. Knisely is affiliated with the Department of Psychiatry, Division of Substance Abuse Medicine, Medical College of Virginia, Richmond, VA. Diane Green is affiliated with the Department of Internal Medicine, Division of Substance Abuse Medicine, Medical College of Virginia, Richmond, VA. Ronald K. Elswick is affiliated with the Department of Biostatistics, Medical College of Virginia, Richmond, VA.

The staff of West 12, Medical College of Virginia Hospital, provided invaluable clinical assistance during this project. Ms. Betty Duke of the Medical College of Virginia Clinical Research Center, provided data management support. Howard P. Roffwarg graciously provided us the use of his normative sleep data from his Sleep Study Unit at the University of Texas Southwestern Medical Center at Dallas. Kenneth Z. Altshuler, MD, Stanton Sharp Chair of Psychiatry at the University of Texas Southwestern Medical Center at Dallas, provided administrative support to Dr. Kowatch during the preparation of this manuscript.

Address reprint requests to: Robert A. Kowatch, MD, Department of Psychiatry, University of Texas Southwestern Medical Center at Dallas, 5323 Harry Hines Blvd, Dallas, TX 75235-9070.

This research reported in this paper was supported by a grant from The Virginia Commonwealth Center For Substance Abuse to Dr. Kowatch.

This was presented as a poster exhibit at the annual meeting of the Association of Professional Sleep Societies, Minneapolis, MN, June 30, 1990.

SUMMARY. We report on nine patients between the ages of 21 and 39 years who were admitted to an inpatient substance abuse treatment unit for cocaine treatment. The patients' sleep was studied in the laboratory for 4 nights during the first week, and 2 nights during the second and third weeks of their hospitalization. Daily mood ratings, cocaine craving scores and sleep logs were also recorded on each patient. During the first week of withdrawal, these patients had a markedly shortened REM latency, an increased REM sleep percentage, a very high REM density and a long total sleep period time. During the third week, REM latencies were very short and total percentage of REM sleep was increased. By week three of withdrawal the sleep continuity pattern was similar to that found in chronic insomnia, with a long sleep latency, an abnormally increased total time awake after sleep onset and a poor sleep efficiency. The subjects' ratings of cocaine craving, total POMS scores and depression fell precipitously after the first week of withdrawal and were at sub-clinical levels by week three of withdrawal.

INTRODUCTION

In patients withdrawing from chronic cocaine use, three phases of abstinence symptoms have been described.[1] The three phases are: (1) crash (1-4 days); (2) withdrawal (1-10 weeks); and (3) extinction (indefinite). Sleep symptoms for the phases are described as insomnia with increased desire to sleep, leading to hypersomnolence during phase one and normalization of sleep early in phase two. Phase two progresses to substantial anhedonia, anxiety, mild dysphoria, anergia and increased cocaine craving. It is during this second phase that most cocaine addicts either obtain more cocaine and begin the binge cycle again, enter into treatment or achieve abstinence on their own. The last phase, extinction, occurs if abstinence from cocaine can be sustained. During this last phase the patient experiences a euthymic mood and episodic cocaine craving.

The sleep patterns of cocaine addicts during the phases of withdrawal have not been extensively studied in the sleep laboratory. Post et al.,[2] administered cocaine in divided doses of 65-200 mg per day to five moderately depressed patients for an average of six days. Cocaine significantly depressed total REM sleep time and total sleep time. Watson et al.,[3] studied the sleep patterns of four individuals withdrawing from 40-200 mg of amphetamines daily for at least five months. During the second through fourth nights of withdrawal, these patients showed an increased amount of REM sleep and an increased percentage of REM sleep. All of these patients became depressed during withdrawal and total sleep time, REM sleep time, and total REMs correlated positively with their depression ratings. Watson et al.,[4] also evaluated the effects of 1-2 grams of cocaine on the sleep of three outpatients described as "recreational" cocaine users. They found that on the night following cocaine use total sleep time was reduced, REM percentage and REM time was reduced, REM latency was lengthened and sleep latency was increased. On the first and second recovery nights, the percentage of REM sleep increased and REM latency was shortened. All of these changes had resolved by the third recovery night.

The purpose of this study was to record the sleep and mood ratings of subjects who were moderately heavy users of cocaine during a drug free withdrawal period.

SUBJECTS AND METHODS

Subjects

Nine patients who were admitted to the inpatient Substance Abuse Unit at the Medical College of Virginia Hospitals for cocaine withdrawal and treatment were recruited for the study. Admission criteria for the study were; diagnosis of cocaine dependence by DSM-III-R criteria;[5] absence of other Axis I psychiatric disorders; not using greater than two marijuana cigarettes/week and or more than the equivalent of four 12 oz. cans of beers/week; no use of psychotropic medication including sedative-hypnotics; no other concurrent substance use other than cocaine; 21-40 years of age; no major medical illness, pregnancy or other primary sleep disorder and the ability to give informed consent.

Procedure

All subjects were screened on the day of admission to determine if they met inclusion criteria for the study and informed consent was obtained. Subjects were paid $10.00 for each nights participation in the study.

All subjects simultaneously participated in a substance abuse treatment program. Subjects were involved in group sessions 5 days a week, daily educational sessions, peer support groups three times a week and individual sessions with a therapist three times a week.

All subjects underwent a physical exam, laboratory tests (complete blood count, electrolytes, liver function studies, serology, HIV antibody test, thyroid function tests, urinalysis and urine drug screens). The majority of subjects had stopped using cocaine one or two days prior to admission. All subjects were required to have a positive urine test for cocaine on admission and a negative test for other substances as per the exclusion criteria. The subjects also submitted random urine toxicologic screens at least twice while enrolled in the study. None of these samples were positive for any substances including cocaine.

All of the subjects were admitted on a Monday and then studied on the next four consecutive nights of that week. Sleep studies were then repeated on Sunday and Monday of weeks two and three of hospitalization.

INSTRUMENTS

On admission, the subjects were interviewed by a psychiatrist and administered the Addiction Severity Index (ASI),[6] a quantitative cocaine inventory which detailed cocaine use for the week prior to admission, a 24 item Hamilton Depression Scale,[7] a Profile of Moods States[8] and a visual-analogue (1-10) cocaine craving scale. Six of the subjects were interviewed a second time, three weeks after admission, by a psychiatrist using the Structured Clinical Interview for DSM-III-R (SCID).[9] Subjects 1, 4, and 7 were interviewed during their second week of hospitalization after they indicated that they would not be staying for the full three week program. Following each nights sleep study at 4 P.M., the subjects were rated using the Hamilton Depression Scale, the POMS and the cocaine craving scale. On non-sleep study days, subjects were rated using a POMS scale and a cocaine craving scale. Subjects were encouraged not to take any daytime naps but, if they did choose to nap, they were asked to record this in a daily sleep log.

Sleep-Recording Methods

Sleep studies were performed in comfortable, private bedrooms. The subjects' skin was cleaned with an abrasive paste and electrodes were applied with collodion to the scalp and adhesive collars to the face. The sleep state was recorded by EEG, electro-oculogram (EOG), and submental chin electromyograms. The EEG consisted of a C4 scalp placement referenced to tied mastoids. The EOG consisted of electrode placements at the outer canthi of the eyes, with each eye derivation referenced to tied mastoids. All electrode impedances were determined to be less than 500 ohms. Filter settings for the EEG and EOG were 0.3 to 70 Hz; the submental chin electromyogram was bipolar, with filter settings of 10 to 90 Hz. Paper speed for all recordings was 10 mm/s. and a 50 micro-volt signal was calibrated to produce a 10-mm deflection at a sensitivity of 5. Respiratory monitoring was done on the first night of the study and consisted of an oral-nasal thermistor airflow monitoring, inductance plethysmography and digital pulse oximetry (Nelcor). After the first night's respiratory monitoring, EEG, EMG, EOG and leg movements were monitored during subsequent recordings. Recordings were made on a sixteen channel polygraph (Grass Model 78-16).

Sleep stages were scored in 30 second epochs according to Rechtschaffen and Kales criteria.[10] All polysomnograms were scored by the same technician who was blind to the subjects diagnosis and who had demonstrated a scoring reliability > 85%. All of the sleep recordings were reviewed by an accredited clinical polysomnographer (R.A.K.) who reviewed the record for sleep apneas, periodic leg movements, sleep and REM latencies. No clinically significant periods of sleep apnea, nocturnal myoclonus or cardiac arrhythmias were seen.

The subjects were scheduled for admittance to the study and treatment program 1-2 weeks prior to actual admission. The majority of subjects binged heavily on cocaine during that week prior to admission and reported sleeping very little during that week. Most of the subjects reported that their usual bedtime for the two week period prior to their admission was between midnight and 3 A.M. and their usual waketime between 9-10 A.M. They had, by virtue of their cocaine use, developed a mild phase delay syndrome of their sleep wake cycle. For the first week in the sleep laboratory subjects were allowed to go to bed when they felt tired and this was usually around 1-2 A.M. Subjects were allowed to awaken spontaneously in the morning and their average wake-up time was 9 A.M though several of the subjects slept to 11 AM during the first two days of withdrawal. By the second week, all of the subjects were going to bed around 11 P.M. and awakening between 7-8 A.M. Subjects' quality of sleep was rated on a standard sleep lab questionnaire after each night's study.

VARIABLES MEASURED

The sleep variables were divided into three groups: sleep continuity, sleep architecture, and REM measures.

Sleep Continuity variables include: *Total recording time:* time in minutes from lights-out to lights-on, including wake time out of bed. *Total sleep period:* time in minutes from sleep onset to wake-up time. *Total sleep time:* minutes of sleep within the total sleep period. *Sleep efficiency:* the ratio of total time asleep to total recording period expressed as a percentage. This measure represents the proportion of the total time available for sleep that is spent in sleep, regardless of whether the sleep occurs before, during, or after the persistent sleep period. *Sleep onset:* the first minute of ten consecutive minutes of stage 1 or greater sleep with no more than two intervening minutes of awake time. *Number of awakenings from sleep within the total sleep period:* An awakening was defined as an EEG arousal lasting 30 seconds or longer. Movement time and out-of-bed times were included in this variable. *Total time awake:* total time awake within the total sleep period. *Rate/hour of sleep awakenings within the total sleep period: rate/hour of sleep stage shifts within the total sleep period.*

Sleep Architecture variables are the percentages of time asleep in the different stages of sleep out of the total sleep period.

REM measures include: *REM latency:* the time from sleep onset to the first 30 second epoch of REM sleep minus any awakenings. *Rapid eye movement period (REMP):* any occurrence of REM sleep lasting for at least two consecutive minutes. Separate REMPs are defined by the occurrence of at least 25 minutes of non-REM staging. A REMP is sometimes composed of several REM fragments separated by less than 25 minutes of non-REM sleep. *Number of REM periods. REMP time:* length of REMP in minutes. *REM activity units:* eye movements per minute of REM, as graded on a scale of 0 to 8 (semi-quantitative). Zero indicates no eye movements; 1 indicates eye movements occupy one-eight (7.5 cms) of the one minute epoch, 2 indicates eye movements occupy 15 cms. of the one minute epoch, etc. *REM activity per period:* sum of REM activity units during a REMP. *REM density per period:* REM activity for a period divided by the actual REM time for that period. *Average REM Density:* sum of all REM densities/period divided by the sum of all REM time across REMPS.

STATISTICAL ANALYSIS

Using the subjects' reports of their last use of cocaine, their exact withdrawal day in relation to their sleep study night was calculated. This value was then used for all subsequent analysis. A control group was not studied, but subjects' sleep variables were compared to normative values provided by Howard P. Roffwarg from the Sleep Study Unit at the University of Texas Southwestern Medical Center at Dallas.[11] These control subjects were all carefully screened for any sleep, medical or psychiatric pathology prior to their inclusion in the normative database and their sleep recordings were scored by strict Rechtschaffen and Kales criteria. There were 51 subjects in this normative group, grouped by age according to decade. Data from these norms in the third decade, ages 20-29, was chosen for the analysis. There were a total of 11 controls in this decade. Scoring methods between our study and the University of Texas at Dallas Sleep Center were the same except for the scoring of rapid eye movement density. Rapid eye movement activity during REM sleep was scored using a 0-8 semi-quantitative scale.[12]

Published norms from the Western Psychiatric Institute and Clinic Sleep Evaluation Center were used for comparison of REM activity and density values.[13]

One sample t-tests were used to compare the subject's mean sleep variables to the norms. Using only the data from the subject group, PROC GLM in SAS was used to apply univariate repeated measure analysis of variance to determine if there was a trend across withdrawal day for each of the sleep variables. Nonparametric indices of partial correlation based on matching was computed between the sleep variables and the daily measures (controlling for withdrawal day) using PROC MATPAR in SAS.

RESULTS

Demographic and clinical characteristics of the nine subjects are presented in Table 1. There were five males and four females, with a mean (± SD) age of 28.5 ± 5.8 years and a range of age from 22 to 39 years. The mean weekly amount of cocaine used in the one week period prior to admission for the subjects was 5.7 g. and their mean (± SD) number of days used in the last week was 4.6 ± 2.1 days. The subjects mean (± SD) duration of cocaine use since first starting to use cocaine was 2.3 ± 1.7 years. The majority of the subjects smoked cocaine free base as their primary route of administration. Values of sleep continuity for the subjects and the normative values are presented in Table 2. During withdrawal the subjects' total sleep period (Fig. 1) and total sleep time increased during weeks one and two. By week three, the subjects' total sleep period and total sleep time were near normal. The subjects' sleep efficiency was poor throughout the study even at week three. Their sleep latency deteriorated across the three week study period. Their total time awake throughout the night also remained elevated throughout the study. These sleep continuity variables revealed that, although the subjects slept longer than would be expected for their age, their sleep was fragmented and of poor quality. By week three, their sleep continuity pattern was similar to that found in chronic insomnia, with a long sleep latency, increased total time awake during the night and a poor sleep efficiency.

The subjects' sleep architecture variables and normative values are presented in Table 3 and revealed an increased percentage of REM sleep (Fig. 2) and a decreased percentage of slow wave sleep (stages 3 & 4). The subjects' REM measures and normative values are presented in Table 4 and showed a shortened REM latency (Fig. 3), increased number of REM periods (Fig. 4), increased REM activity and increased REM density (Fig. 5). A univariate repeated measures analysis of variance did not find any statistically significant difference in the sleep variables across time.

The means of the sleep reports of the quality of sleep across the withdrawal period taken after each night's sleep recording are presented in Figure 6. During the first three days of withdrawal, subjects reported "sleeping worse than usual" but later reported that the quality of their sleep was "the same as usual."

The subjects' subjective ratings of cocaine craving, total POMS scores and depression ratings fell precipitously after the first week of withdrawal (Figures 7 & 8). McNair et al. reported a mean total score on the POMS of 8.4 for a group of 113 college males.[14] Both the total Hamilton score and the cocaine craving rating showed changes that were statistically significant over time ($p < .01$) using repeated measures ANOVA. Indices of correlation between the Hamilton scores, the total POMS score, the POMS subscale scores, the cocaine craving scores and the sleep variables were low except for REM latency, which correlated significantly ($p < .001$) with the mean cocaine craving score (index of correlation = +.34), the mean Hamilton score (index of correlation = +.32) and the depression subscale of the POMS (index of correlation = +.24)

Subjects who had smoked cocaine free-base, coughed frequently throughout the night during the first week's recordings. No cardiac arrhythmias or significant periods of either obstructive or central sleep apnea were seen during any of the sleep study nights.

COMMENT

Gawin and Kleber's observations that a period of hypersomnolence lasting up to four days following cocaine withdrawal was partially confirmed by this study. A period of hypersomnolence was observed through withdrawal day nine but was not present by day

Table 1. Subject Characteristics

Patient Number	Age, Years	Gender	Hollingshead Social Class	Education, Years
1	24	M	IV	10
2	28	M	III	14
3	22	F	V	11
4	22	F	V	12
5	39	F	V	9
6	25	M	IV	12
7	33	M	IV	14
8	32	M	IV	12
9	32	F	V	12
Mean + S.D.	**28.5 + 5.8**		**IV**	**11.8 + 1.6**

15. Our subjects' sleep, however, had not "normalized" after the first week of withdrawal as Gawin and Kleber had reported in their 30 subjects. Rather, our subjects showed a pattern consistent with insomnia by week three of withdrawal, with a prolonged sleep latency, a poor sleep efficiency and increased awake time throughout the night. Although the subjects' total sleep time was prolonged during the first week of withdrawal, the quality of their sleep, both objectively and subjectively was poor. This result was surprising since our population was roughly equivalent to Gawin and Kleber's

Years of Cocaine Use	Grams Used In Past Week	Days Used In Past Week	Route of Administration
3	17.5	7	Intravenous
2	1.5	3	FB
1	3	4	FB
1	9	7	FB
3	3.5	7	FB
0.5	5	5	FB
3	7.5	4	FB
6	1	1	FB
1	3.5	3	FB
2.3 + 1.7	**5.7 + 5.1**	**4.6 + 2.1**	**FB**

FB = Smoked

population in relation to age and estimated use of cocaine. Their findings were based upon semi-structured interviews which may not have been sensitive enough to elicit the same sleep patterns we observed.

The persistence of REM abnormalities over the three week study period is consistent with the sleep studies in patients with major depression: shortened REM latency and a high REM density.[15] There was a low correlation between these REM measures and the subjects' mood and cocaine craving ratings.

The neurochemical effects of chronic cocaine use and subsequent withdrawal are complex and poorly understood. A preliminary study

Table 2. Sleep Continuity Measures (Mean sleep variable + S.D.)

	Normative Values	Subject Values Week One		
Withdrawal Day		2	3	4
Number of subjects	11	6	7	9
Total recording time, min	411.1+40.1	522.66+134.6	469.57+80*	495.66+114.9*
Total sleep period, min	395.7+41.5	499.66+126.3	440.14+80.8	453.4+134.3
Total sleep time, min	379.7+41.7	457.16+100.7	417.85+79.3	428.88+128.2
Sleep efficiency, %	92.4	88	89.2	85.8
Sleep latency, min	13.7+12.7	15.5+16.3	25.5+22.9	27.3+27.4
Total time awake, min.	15.8+7.1	49.2+29.1*	47.5+32.2*	61.5+48.5*

*One-sample t-test yielded P<.05

**One-sample t-test yielded P<.01

Table 3. Sleep Architecture Measures (Mean sleep variable + S.D.)

	Normative Values	Subject Values Week One		
Withdrawal Day		2	3	4
Number of subjects	11	6	7	9
% of stage 1 sleep	8.2+2.7	5.6+3.0	6.4+3.0	9.4+5.2
% of stage 2 sleep	57.5+4.7	59.3+10.3	61.4+7.7	54.3+18.6
% of stage 3 sleep	9.0+3.3	3.5+3.5**	3.0+3.21**	2.1+2.7**
% of stage 4 sleep	3.7+2.9	0	0	0.1+0.3**
% of stage REM sleep	17.5+4.1	23.2+7.9	23.8+7.8	21.2+4.5*
% of stage 0 + movement time	4.0+1.8	4.6+3.6	4.5+2.5	4.2+1.7

*One-sample t-test yielded P<.05

**One-sample t-test yielded P<.01

Table 2 (continued)

		Week Two		Week Three		
5	6	8	9	15	16	17
7	3	5	5	4	3	3
504.14+87.0*	436.33+98.0	477.20+21.2**	497.80+37.0**	458.75+42.4	466.0+7.5*	373.0+23.5
480+99.5	418.33+84.3	453.40+20.3**	471.80+36.8**	400.70+90.6	429.66+46.8	331.3+52.9
442.28+111.3	395.33+87.0	439.60+17.6**	448.00+57.6*	379.25+87.5	420.66+48.4	319.6+49.5
87	90.6	92.6	90	82	90	86.3
20.7+24.2	15.3+10.2	22.4+19.8	24.6+14.3	45.0+40.7	35.3+45.6	39.0+47.0
59.7+32.3*	39.6+12.2	36.2+20.3	46.9+27.1	77.3+53.4	41.6+44.1	48.3+36.0

Table 3 (continued)

		Week Two		Week Three		
5	6	8	9	15	16	17
7	3	5	5	4	3	3
7.0+2.3	9.0+1.0	6.4+3.5	9.0+2.2	7.2+1.7	4.6+2.5	5.6+2.0
56.5+6.3	60.3+5.0	61.2+4.6	58.6+7.0	62.2+6.8	65.6+2.3	67.0+5.0
5.8+6.2	0.6+0.5*	3.6+6.0	3.6+5.1	6.2+6.1	2.6+4.6	3.0+1.7*
0.14+0.3**	0	0	0	0.25+0.5*	0	0
22.0+4.5*	24.3+2.0	25.8+7.1*	23.2+2.7*	19.2+6.3	25.3+4.1	20.0+5.5
6.7+6.8	4.6+1.5	2.8+1.3	5.0+5.0	5.0+4.7	2.3+0.5*	3.0+1.0

FIGURE 1. Total sleep period in minutes per withdrawal day. Subjects' mean values (± S.D.) as compared to age matched normative mean value (± S.D.).; *indicates $p < .05$,; **indicates $p < .01$.

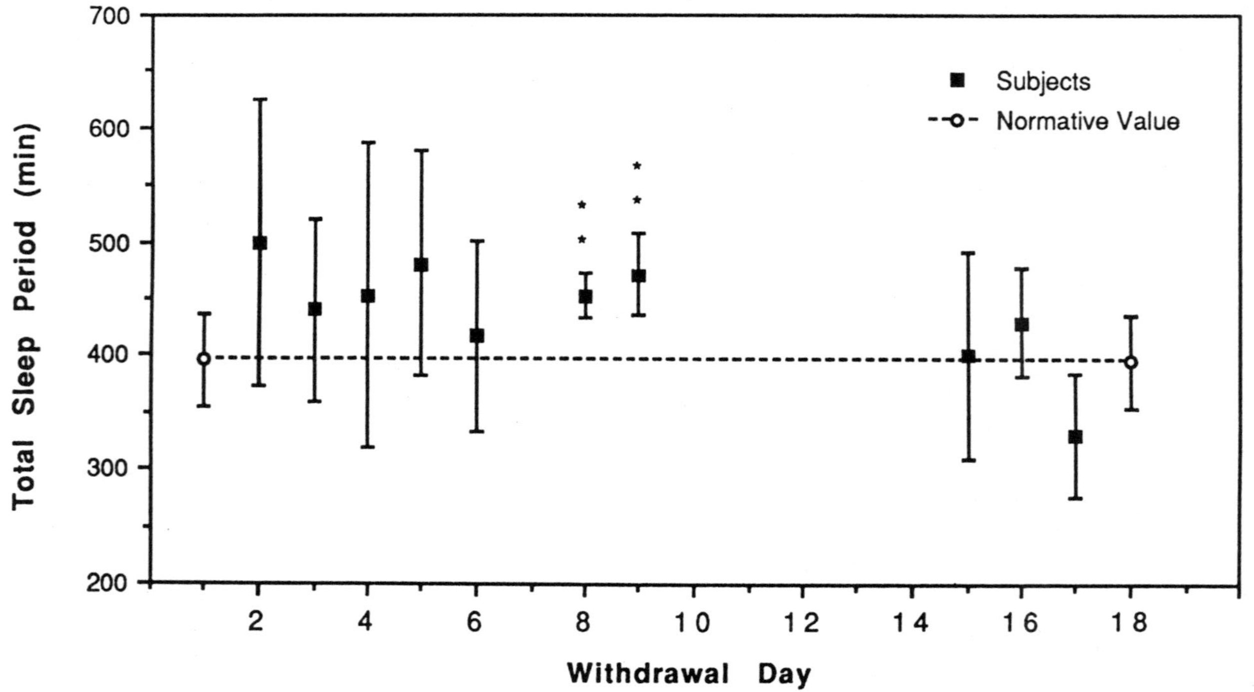

FIGURE 2. Percentage of rapid eye movement (REM) sleep/total sleep period per withdrawal day. Subjects' mean values (± S.D.) as compared to age matched normative mean value (± S.D.).; *indicates $p < .05$,; **indicates $p < .01$.

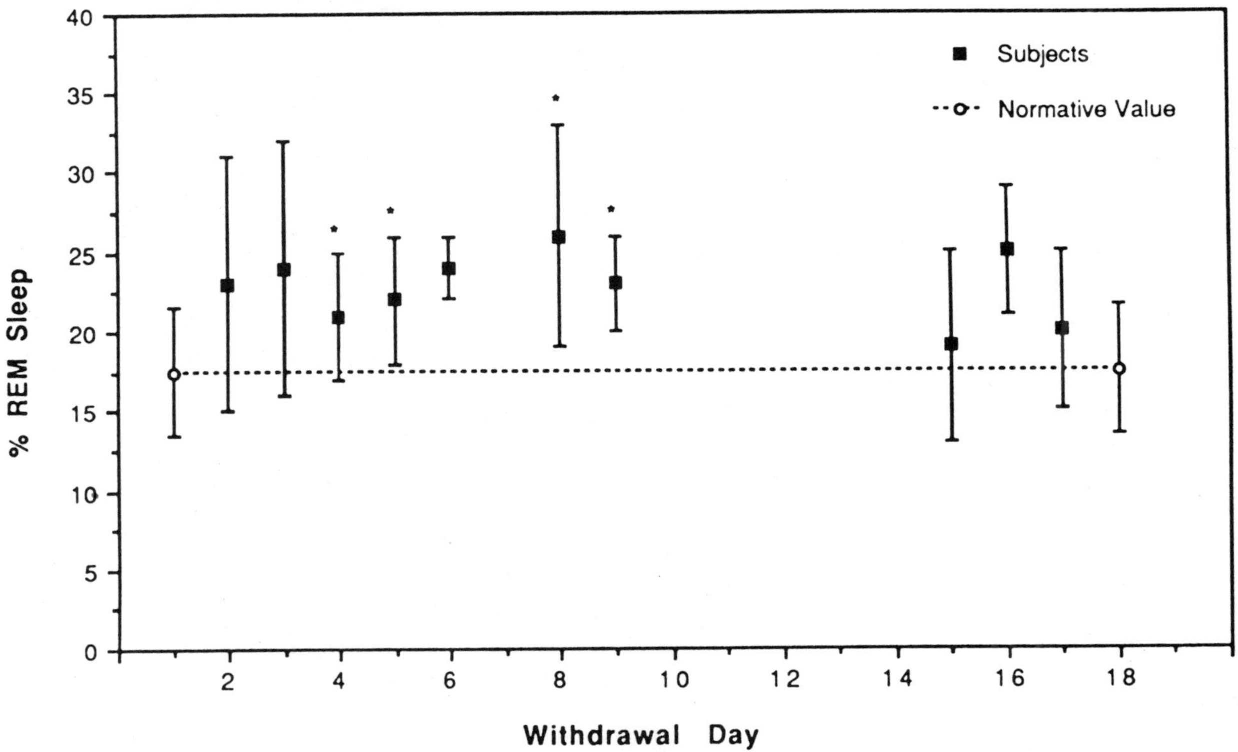

Table 4. REM Sleep Measures (Mean sleep variable + S.D.)

	Normative Values	Subject Values Week One		
Withdrawal Day		2	3	4
Number of subjects	11	6	7	9
REM Measures				
REM latency, min	85+15.1	55.4+41	74.1+25	68.7+45
Number of REM Periods	3.7+0.81	4.0+0.6	4.4+0.5**	4.4+1.4
REM activity, units	79.8+32.9	179.75+124.6	179.9+104.1*	158.3+94.8*
REM density	0.87+.24	1.70+0.9	1.75+0.9*	1.89+1.1*

*One-sample t-test yielded P<.05

**One-sample t-test yielded P<.01

examined the effects of self-administered cocaine in rats and found decreased dopamine and serotonin levels with no change in norepinephrine levels.[16] These decreased serotonin levels could account for the picture of insomnia that we observed in our subjects, as lesions of the dorsal raphe nucleus that contain serotonergic neurons produce profound insomnia in animals.[17] The increased percentage of REM sleep, increased REM density and shortened time to the first REM period that were observed in this study, are suggestive of a heightened pressure for REM sleep during cocaine withdrawal. Cholinergic stimulation appears to trigger REM sleep in both humans and animals as arecoline, a specific muscarinic agonist, triggers REM sleep.[18] Recently, it has been suggested that in addition to cocaine's effects upon the catecholamine system, cocaine also decreases acetylcholine release by activating dopamine receptors on cholinergic neurons.[19] During cocaine withdrawal, an increased level of acetylcholine might occur as a result of suppression during active cocaine use. This would explain the increased "pressure" (increased REM percent, shortened REM latency and increased REM density) for REM sleep that was observed in the present study. The fact that the subjects' REM latency remained shortened at week three was curious and suggests that the time course for neurochemical recovery following chronic cocaine use persists for at least three weeks.

		Week Two		Week Three		
5	6	8	9	15	16	17
7	3	5	5	4	3	3
64.8+15**	60.6+15	47.8+25.4*	52.0+23.6*	61.0+23.1	62.3+14.7	54.6+9.8*
4.4+0.5*	4.3+1.1	4.6+0.5*	4.4+0.5*	4.0+1.8	4.3+0.5	3.3+0.5
162.1+73.5*	125.3+20.4	123.6+70.6	159.9+77.6	98.1+44.2	134.7+127.6	82.7+27.5
1.70+0.6**	1.27+0.1	1.11+0.6	1.46+0.7	1.5+0.5	1.16+0.8	1.25+0.3

The results of this study are limited due to the small number of subjects per withdrawal day and the large individual differences that were observed between subjects' sleep recordings. In future studies, it would be important to include a larger sample size, extend the study period, control for the subject's last use of cocaine and attempt to schedule their sleep studies around this time. It would also be important to determine if there is any relationship between the degree of sleep disruption seen during the withdrawal period and later relapse.

Various medications have been studied as treatments for cocaine withdrawal; desipramine, lithium, bromocriptine and prolixin.[20] Desipramine suppresses REM sleep but worsens sleep continuity and would not seem to be a good choice to treat the sleep disturbance observed during the withdrawal period.[21] Neuroleptics tend to decrease wakefulness, increase slow wave sleep and have variable effects upon REM sleep depending upon how specific their dopaminergic effects are.[22] Alprazolam, a triazolobenzodiazepine, has been shown to both suppress REM sleep and improve sleep continuity measures.[23] For these reasons, it may be a useful drug to study in treating the sleep disturbance seen during cocaine withdrawal.

FIGURE 3. Rapid eye movement (REM) latency, corrected values per withdrawal day. Subjects' mean values (± S.D.) as compared to age matched normative mean value (± S.D.).; *indicates $p < .05$,; **indicates $p < .01$.

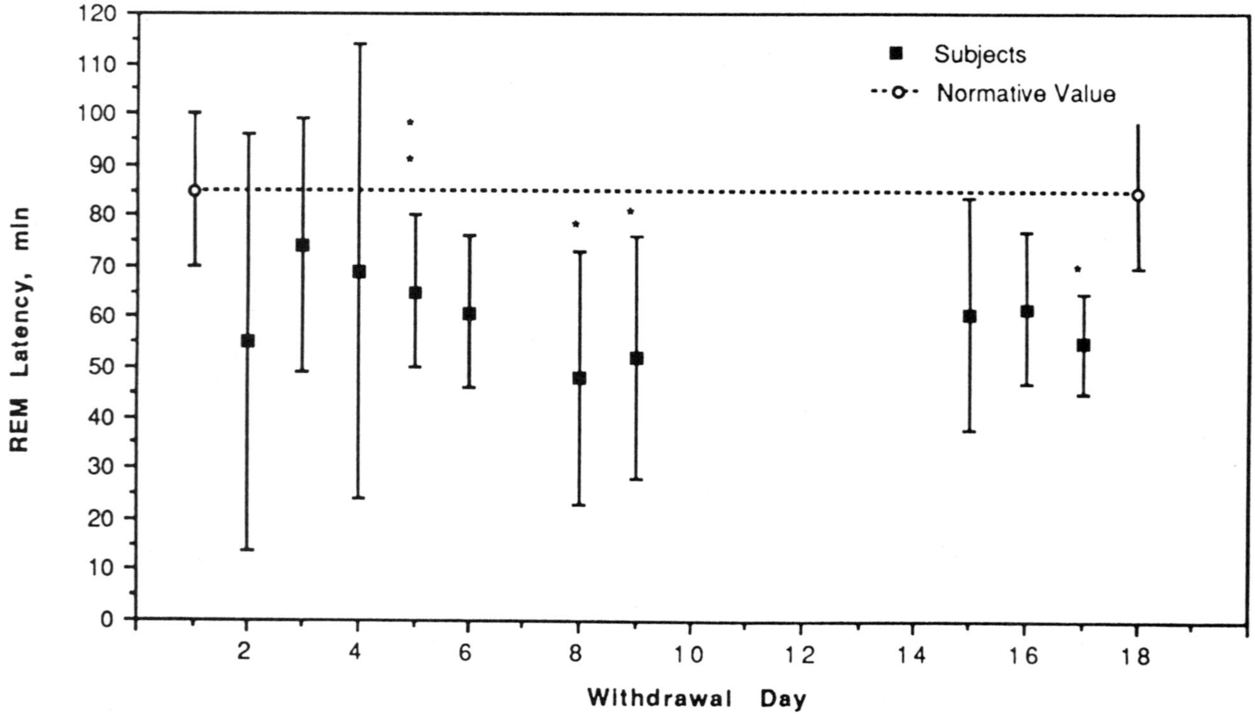

FIGURE 4. Number of rapid eye movement (REM) periods (25 minute rule) per withdrawal day. Subjects' mean values (± S.D.) as compared to age matched normative mean value (± S.D.).; *indicates $p < .05$,; **indicates $p < .01$.

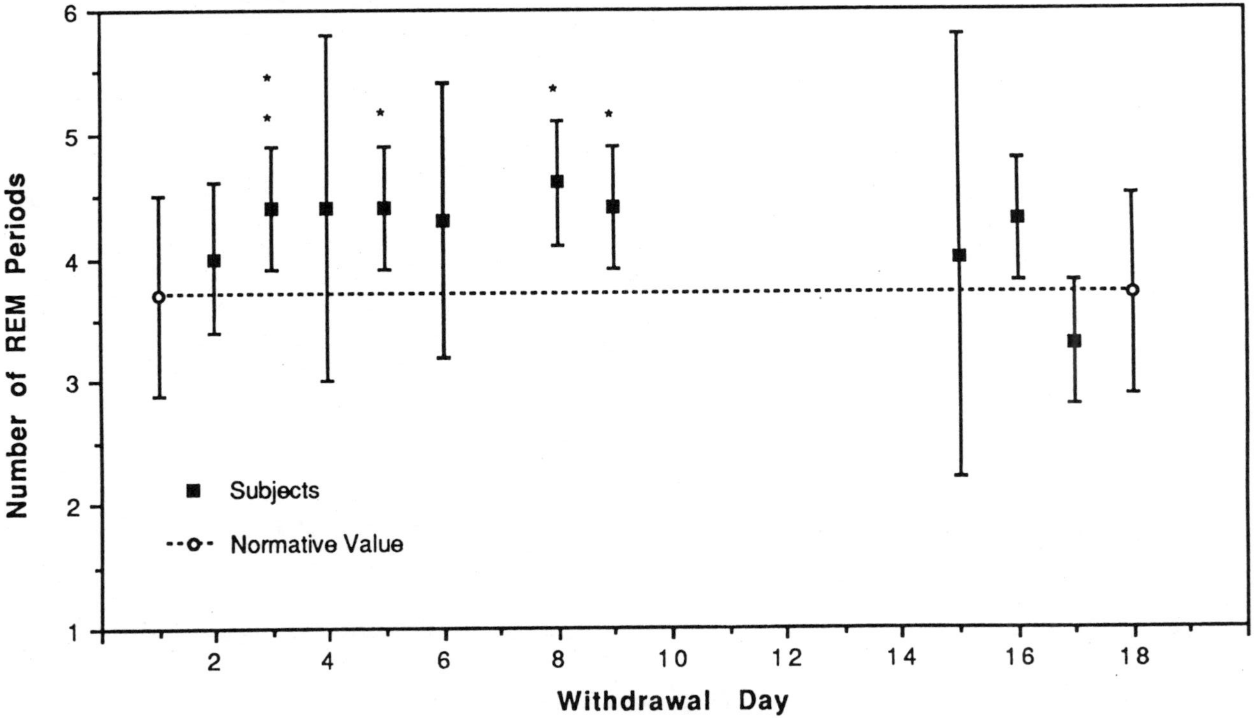

FIGURE 5. Rapid eye movement (REM) density per withdrawal day. Subjects' mean values (± S.D.) as compared to age matched normative mean value (± S.D.).; *indicates $p < .05$,; **indicates $p < .01$.

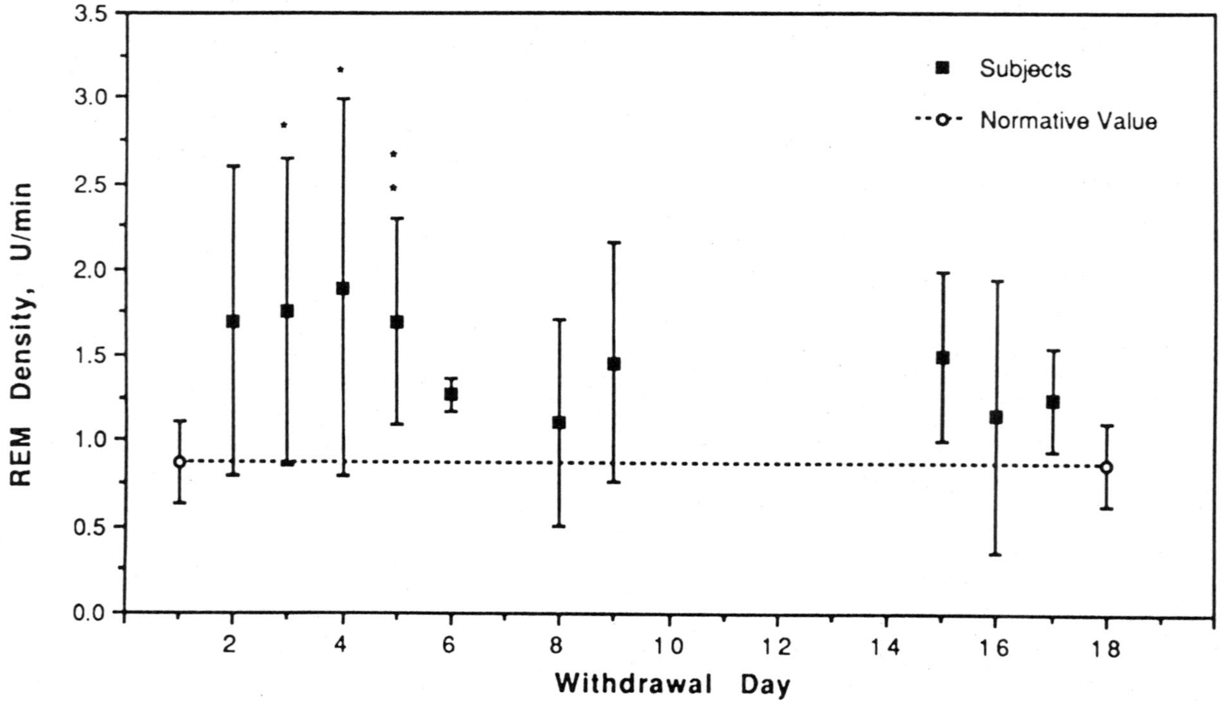

FIGURE 6. Mean rating of sleep quality after each recording night in the laboratory; rated immediately upon arising. (1 = much worse than usual, 2 = worse than usual, 3 = same as usual, 4 = better than usual)

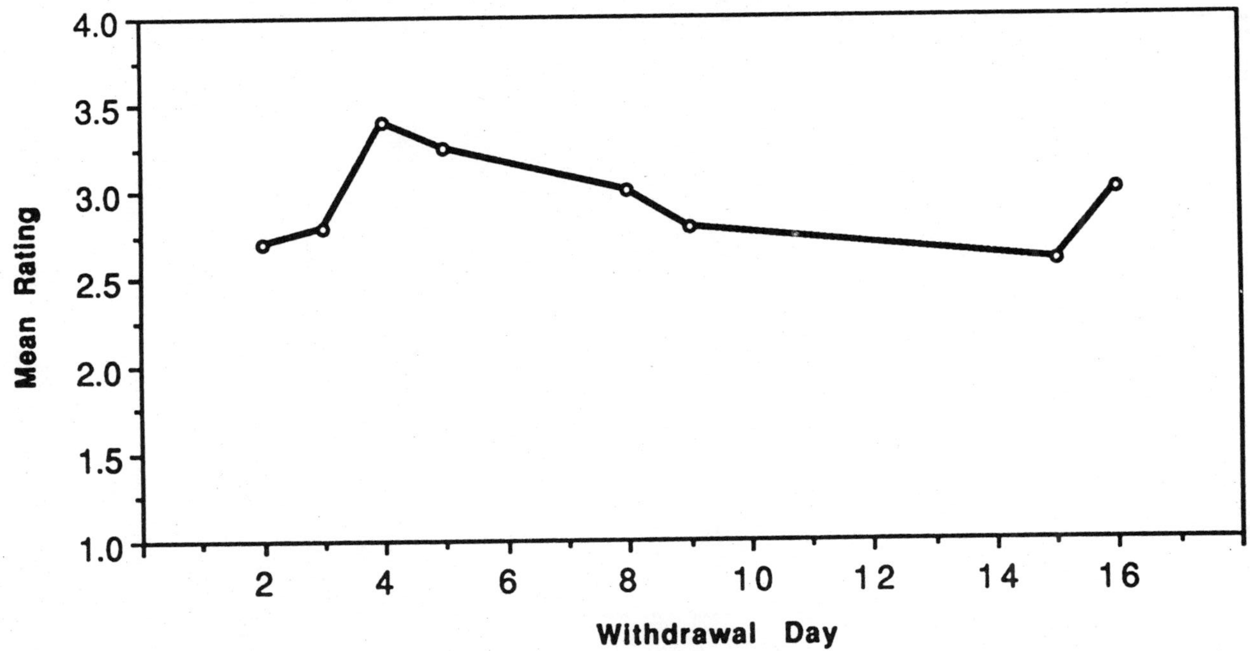

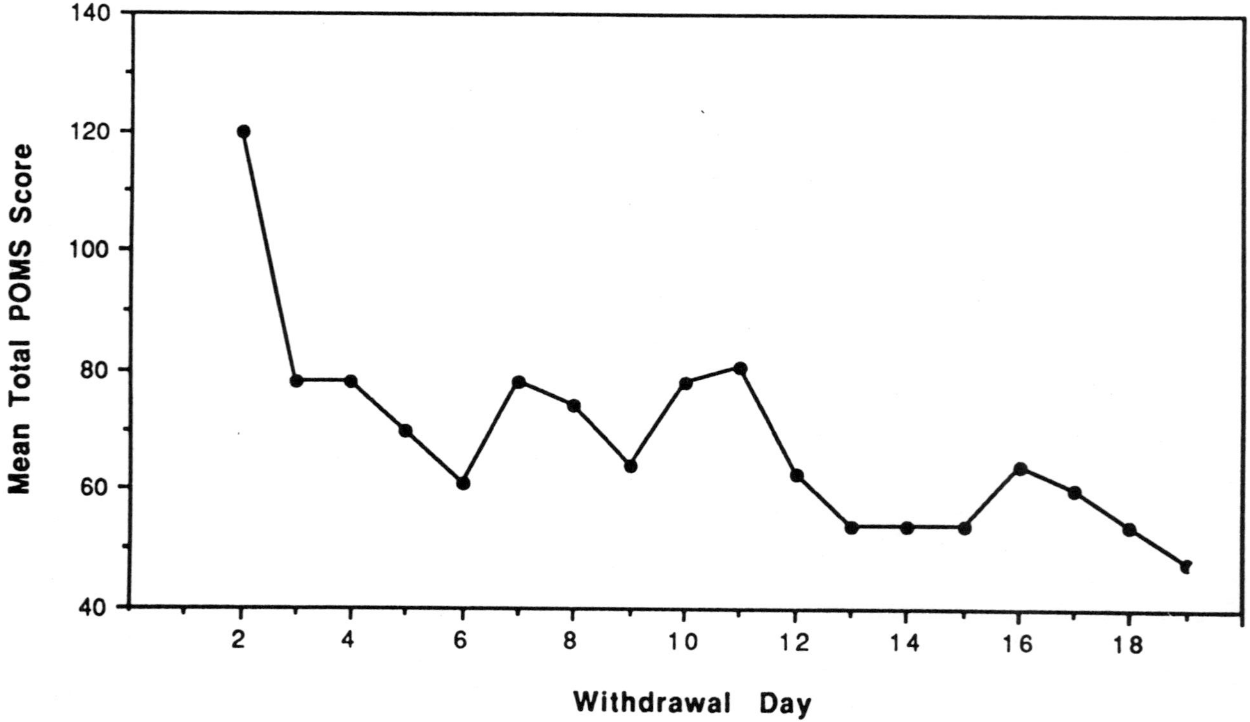

FIGURE 7. Mean total POMS score (vigor subscale weighted negatively) per withdrawal day.

FIGURE 8. Mean cocaine craving and Hamilton Depression Rating Scores per withdrawal day; cocaine craving score: 1-10 visual analogue scale with 10 indicating severe craving; 24 item Hamilton Depression Scale.

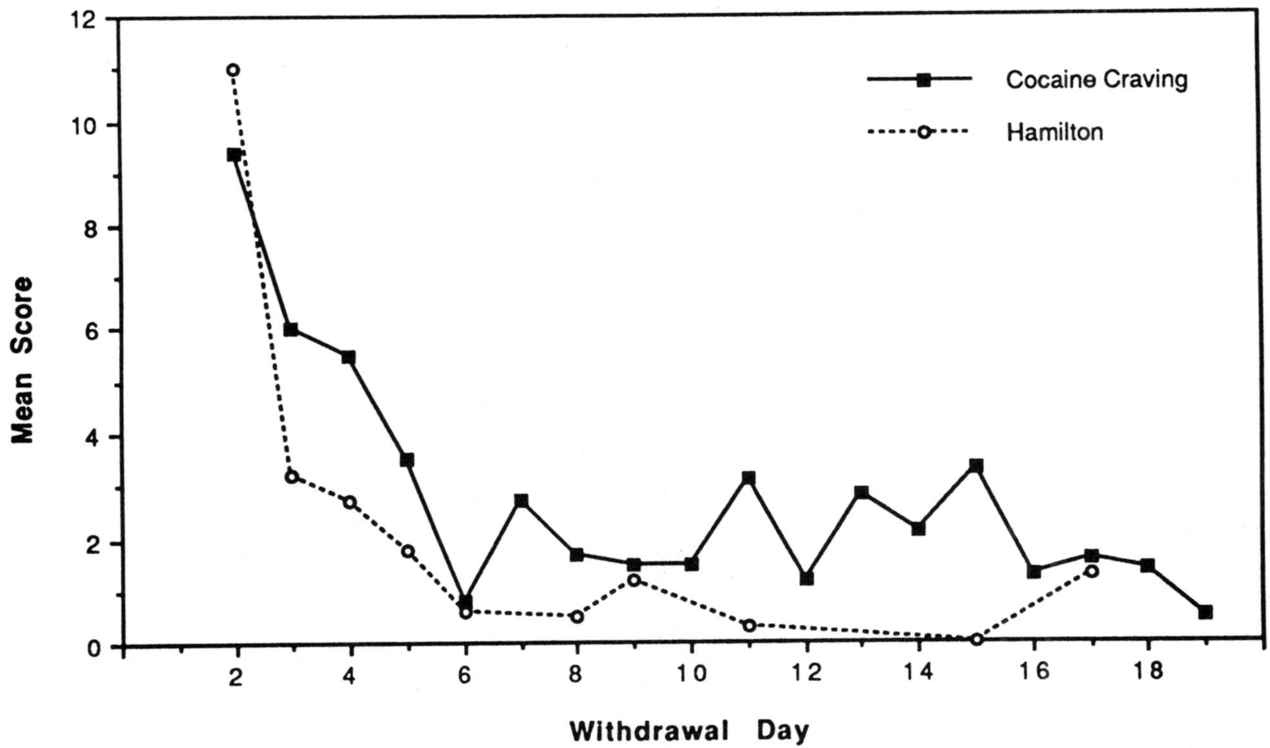

REFERENCES

1. Gawin, FH & Kleber, HD: Abstinence symptomatology and psychiatric diagnosis in cocaine abusers. Arch Gen Psychiatry, 1986; 43:107-113.

2. Post RM, Gillin JC, Wyatt RJ et al: The effect of orally administered cocaine on sleep of depressed patients. Psychopharmacology, 1974; 3:7;59-66.

3. Watson R, Hartman E, Schildkraut JJ: Amphetamine withdrawal in affective state, sleep patterns, and MHPG excretion. Am J Psychiatry, 1972, 129:263-9.

4. Watson R, Bakos L, Compton P, Byck R & Gawin F. Cocaine use and withdrawal: The effect on' sleep and mood. Sleep Research, 1989; 8:83.

5. American Psychiatric Association Committee on Nomenclature and Statistics: Diagnostic and Statistical Manual of Mental Disorders, ed 3, revised. Washington, D.C., American Psychiatric Association, 1987.

6. McClellan MT, Luborsky L, Cacciola J, McGahan P & O'Brien CP. Guide To The Addiction Severity Index: Background, Administration & Field Testing Results. Washington, D.C.: National Institute of Drug Abuse, 1988.

7. Hamilton M. Development of a rating scale for primary depressive illness. Brit J Soc Psychol, 6:278-296, 1967.

8. McNair DM, Lorr M, Droppleman LF. EDITS manual for the Profile of Moods States. San Diego: Educational Testing Service, 1981.

9. Spitzer RL, Williams JBL, Gibbon M: Structured Clinical Interview for DSM III-R. New York, Biometrics Research Division, New York State Psychiatric Institute, 1987.

10. Rechtschaffen A, Kales AA, eds. A manual of standardized terminology, techniques and scoring system for sleep stages of human subjects. University of California at Los Angles: Brain Information Service/Brain Research Institute, 1968.

11. Roffwarg, HP, Rush, J, Carpenter, G, Giles, D, Fairchild, C. Normal sleep reconsidered: The effects of age on sleep structure in a "true" normal population. Presented at Sleep Research Society, June 1, 1985. Toronto, Canada.

12. Taska LS and Kupfer DJ. Sleep Scoring Manual, 1987.

13. Kupfer, DJ, Ulrich, RF, Coble, PA, Jarrett, DB, Grochocinski, VJ, Doman, J, Matthews, G & Borbely, AA. Electroencephalographic sleep of younger depressives: Comparison with normals. 1985; Arch Gen Psychiatry 42:806-810.

14. McNair DM, Lorr M, Droppleman LF. EDITS manual for the Profile of Moods States. San Diego: Educational Testing Service, 1981.

15. Reynolds, C.F., Kupfer, D.J.: State-of the art review, Sleep research in affective illness: State of the art circa, 1987; Sleep 1987, Vol 10, No. 3; 199-215.

16. Bozarth MA. New perspectives on cocaine addiction: recent findings from animal research. Can J Physiolo Pharmacol 1989;67: 1158-1167.

17. Gaillard JM, Nicholson AN & Pascoe PA. Neurotransmitter Systems. In Textbook of Sleep Disorders Medicine, Krieger (eds) 1989, p 206.

18. Gaillard JM, Nicholson AN & Pascoe PA. Neurotransmitter Systems. In Textbook of Sleep Disorders Medicine, Krieger (eds) 1989, p 203.

19. Hurd YL, Weiss F, Koob G & Ungerstedt U. The influence of cocaine self-administered on in vivo dopamine and acetylcholine neurotransmission in rat caudate-putamen. Neurosci Lett, 1990; 109:227-233.

20. Gawin FH & Ellinwood EH. Cocaine and other stimulants: Actions, abuse and treatment. N Engl J Med, 1988; 318:18;1173-1182.

21. Shipley JE, Kupfer DJ, Griffin SJ, Dealy RS, Coble PA, McEachran AB, Grochinski VJ, Ulrich R & Perel JM. Comparison of effects of desipramine and amitriptyline on EEG sleep of depressed patients. Psychopharmacology. 1985; 85:14-22.

22. Nicholson AN, Bradley CM & Pascoe PA. Medications: Effect on sleep and Wakefulness. In Textbook of Sleep Disorders Medicine, Krieger (eds) 1989, p 228.

23. Hubain PP, Castro P, Mesters P, De Maertlaer V & Mendlewicz. Alprazalom and amitriptyline in the treatment of major depressive disorder: a double-blind clinical and sleep EEG study. J Affective Disord, 1990; 18:67-73.

Neuropsychiatric Effects of Cocaine: SPECT Measurements

Bruce L. Miller, MD
Ismael Mena, MD
Robert Giombetti, MD
Javier Villanueva-Meyer, MD
A. H. Djenderedjian, MD

SUMMARY. Cocaine causes serious neurologic and neuropsychiatric complications. Cocaine-induced seizures are common and appear to be due to the local anaesthetic actions of this compound. Cocaine induced stroke has varied mechanisms. With ischemic stroke there is severe vasospasm induced by rises in brain catecholamines. These changes can persist for many weeks and can be demonstrated using single-photon emission computerized tomography (SPECT). In many patients with psychiatric symptoms such as psychosis or mania, SPECT demonstrates similar changes in cerebral blood flow. In fact, some of the psychiatric symptoms induced by cocaine may be due to decreases in cerebral blood flow. In cocaine abuse, treatment strategies based on decreasing cerebral vasospasm need to be developed.

INTRODUCTION

Cocaine use has reached epidemic proportions with over 6 million users estimated in the United States in 1990.[1] The psychiatric

---

Bruce L. Miller is affiliated with the Department of Neurology; Ismael Mena is affiliated with the Department of Radiology; Robert Giombetti is affiliated with the Department of Neurology; Javier Villanueva-Meyer is affiliated with the Department of Radiology; and A. H. Djenderedjian is affiliated with the Department of Psychiatry, all at the Harbor-UCLA Medical Center, Torrance, CA.

Please address all correspondence to: Bruce L. Miller, MD, Department of Neurology, B-4, Harbor-UCLA Medical Center, Torrance, CA 90509.

sequelae of acute and chronic cocaine intoxication are well recognized and have been documented with comprehensive research reports,[2] news specials and television documentaries. Similarly, the cardiac toxicity of cocaine has been studied. (See Nademanee in this volume.)[3] However, there have been surprisingly few clinical investigations that have detailed the neurologic complications of cocaine abuse. Similarly, there is little on the patho-mechanisms for these neurological toxicities.

Recent work has demonstrated that the neurological sequelae are largely due to the effects cocaine on cerebral vessels. With the advent of high resolution single photon emission computerized tomography (SPECT), it has become possible to demonstrate in-vivo changes in cerebral blood flow associated with cocaine abuse.

We will briefly describe the neurologic and neuropsychiatric complications seen with cocaine intoxication and discuss the possible mechanisms for these clinical changes. Also, we will review the abnormalities in cerebral blood flow that we have demonstrated in cocaine abusers with Single Photon Emission Computerized Tomography (SPECT). The value of SPECT in the diagnosis and treatment of cocaine intoxication is discussed.

MECHANISMS OF ACTION FOR COCAINE

Research into cocaine within psychiatry has focused on changes in neurotransmitters induced by cocaine abuse. Acutely, cocaine will block re-uptake of brain catecholamines[2] and the "euphoria" associated with cocaine is probably secondary to increased activity in the central dopaminergic reward pathways.[4] The increase in brain catecholamines caused by cocaine not only induces euphoria, but may also account for some of the toxicities of the drug. The chronic use of cocaine causes potentially reversible decreases in D-2 receptor density, which may be linked to the depression seen in these patients.[5] Also, increases in catecholamines can lead to severe vasospasm in both peripheral and cerebral vessels. Finally, cocaine acts as a local anaesthetic which may account for some of its toxicities.

With the increased central and peripheral activity of dopamine and norepinephrine, hypertension, tachycardia, and excitation are seen. With higher doses, hyperthermia, acidosis, seizures, cardiovascular collapse and death occur. With "crack" cocaine, lethal dosages are easily and unpredictably achieved. The widespread availability of crack probably accounts for the epidemic of stroke and seizures in cocaine users that has occurred over the past few years in urban medical centers.[6,7,8]

In an animal study, the mean lethal dosage of intravenous cocaine was 22 mg/kg.[9] Pretreatment with beta-blockers partially blocked cardiovascular effects but did not change the lethal dosage. Similarly, blocking acidosis did not change morbidity. Conversely, making animals hypothermic prior to treatment with cocaine lead to a doubling of the mean lethal dosage. Pretreating with chlorpromazine blocked hyperthermia and acidosis and increased the dosage at which toxicity occurred. Hyperthermia and hyperthermia-induced seizures appeared to be the main cause for death. Surprisingly, cardiovascular mechanisms were less important.

This work has potentially important clinical implications that have been incompletely explored. In most emergency room settings a systematized approach to massive cocaine overdose is needed. However, double-blinded studies using dopamine blockade and/or hypothermia are needed. Also, as will be later described, some of the toxicities associated with cocaine are due to spasm of cerebral vessels. To date, no studies have been performed to determine whether drugs that decrease cerebral vasospasm will improve clinical symptoms. Unfortunately, medical approaches for the treatment of cocaine toxicity have been largely neglected.

NEUROLOGICAL COMPLICATIONS OF COCAINE

At Harbor-UCLA we have seen an epidemic of seizures in young people using cocaine.[7] Both focal and generalized seizures occurred although generalized seizures were more common. Many cocaine abusers do not seek medical attention following a seizure so that the prevalence of cocaine induced seizures is far higher than estimates from emergency room admissions.

Like other local anesthetics, cocaine lowers the seizure threshold.[10] The changes in central catecholamines that are associated with cocaine abuse may also be partially responsible for the lowered seizure threshold. Cocaine induced seizures are typically generalized although focal seizures also occur.[7] If a post-ictal electroencephalogram is normal, chronic treatment with anticonvulsants is not advised. However, focal seizures should stimulate a search for focal brain disease.

In some instances the focal seizures are probably due to focal brain ischemia caused by vasoconstriction of cerebral vessels. Kindling of a seizure focus has been hypothesized to occur as a complication of cocaine,[11] although further work in this area is needed. Benzodiazepines and or phenobarbital[10] should be used to treat cocaine induced status epilepticus, a rare complication of cocaine abuse.

Cerebral ischemia is common with cocaine. At Harbor-UCLA medical center we described 9 individuals with cocaine-induced stroke.[7] The incidence of cocaine induced stroke continues to be high at Harbor-UCLA, and in the month of July 1990 eight patients were evaluated by the neurology service due to stroke or transient ischemic attacks associated with cocaine abuse (Miller BL, personal communication). Sometimes stroke occurs in the first time user and we have described spinal cord vascular infarction with permanent guadriplegia in one such patient.[7] Similarly, transient ischemic attacks, cortical, brainstem and basal ganglia stroke occur, sometimes in first time users.[6,7,8,12]

In the majority of individuals with cocaine-induced ischemic stroke there are no known risk factors for the cerebrovascular disease and there is no way of predicting those patients who will have a neurologic complication while abusing cocaine. With some cases of stroke angiography shows evidence for a vasculitis, although, often it is normal.[7,12] A recent report shows that cocaine can induce a granulomatous angiitis.[13] A cocaine-induced vasculitis could lead to cerebral ischemia lasting for many months after the cocaine use had been discontinued. As will be shown, cerebrovascular spasm may occur for many days after cocaine blood levels have returned to normal.

The management of cocaine-induced ischemic stroke is similar to management of stroke from other causes. Because many of these individuals are in their teens, twenties and thirties a search for a treatable etiology should always be instituted. In many cases angiography will be necessary. In the future it will be important to determine whether therapies designed to decrease cerebral vascular spasm will be effective.

Also common with cocaine abuse is subarachnoid or parenchymal brain hemorrhage. In approximately one-half of these patients there is an underlying arteriovenous malformation or a berry aneurysm shown at angiography.[7,12] It is hypothesized that the hypertension associated with cocaine precipitates hemorrhage in congenitally abnormal vessels. In others the angiogram is normal. With some cases of cocaine-induced subarachnoid hemorrhage, abnormal vessels are probably small and are obliterated with the hemorrhage. In other cases, it is possible that cocaine induces hemorrhage within previously normal vessels.

SPECT CHANGES WITH COCAINE ABUSE: NEUROLOGIC COMPLICATIONS

Recent developments in technology have occurred that allow non-invasive measurements of cerebral blood flow (CBF) with single photon emission computerized tomography (SPECT). With the advent of better brain perfusion agents such as ^{99}Technetium-HMPAO (HMPAO),[14] and improvements in rotating gamma-cameras, quantitative images of cerebral blood flow can now be generated. With the rotating gamma-cameras, a resolution of 16-20 mm is possible with HMPAO (Ceretec). At some institutions, including our own, brain dedicated SPECT systems with multi-ring detectors obtain a resolution of 7-9 mm using compounds such as HMPAO. With these brain-dedicated systems the investigator can obtain an absolute quantitative image of cerebral blood flow with ^{133}Xenon.

At Harbor-UCLA medical center we have studied over 30 patients with acute cocaine intoxication using SPECT. The majority were admitted for neurological symptoms including transient ischemic attack (TIA), ischemic stroke, brain hemorrhage, focal and generalized seizures and migraine headache. In addition, some patients with "purely" psychiatric symptoms including mania, psychosis and depression were studied.

SPECT studies of patients with cocaine precipitated stroke have shown decreased perfusion in the brain regions that correspond to the clinical syndrome. Every patient with focal motor or focal sensory symptoms had focal hypoperfusion in the contralateral hemisphere demonstrated with SPECT. The focal hypoperfusion tended to occur earlier than changes on computerized axial tomography (CT) or magnetic resonance imaging (MRI) and areas of hypoperfusion were larger than the area of infarction seen on MRI. (See Figures 1 and 2). In a few patients CT and MRI stayed normal while SPECT demonstrated hypoperfusion that corresponded to a clinical deficit.

In addition, multiple scalloped areas of diminished perfusion were seen in the areas surrounding the ventricles and in deep portions of the brain[15,16] (See Figure 3). The clinical sequelae of these deep and superficial areas of hypoperfusion are unknown but they occurred in over 80% of the patients evaluated with cocaine intoxication.[15,16] In those with ischemic stroke these changes were more severe, although, in patients with "purely" psychiatric symptoms such as mania, depression or psychosis scalloping also occurred.

The scalloping seen in cocaine abusers is an unusual SPECT finding. However, we have seen a similar pattern in patients with lupus cerebral vasculitis (Giombetti R, personal communication). It appears that SPECT can demonstrate small vessel hypoperfusion and that the scalloping seen with SPECT represents decreased blood flow in vascular regions that are most severely affected by cocaine. There is a predilection for hypoperfusion to occur within white matter in the periventricular regions.

This SPECT "fingerprint" of cocaine intoxication has been helpful in the diagnosis and management of patients with neurologic symptoms. Many abusers will deny use of the drug and if they are admitted several days after the initial use of cocaine, urine toxicology may return to normal. Scalloping tends to persist for days to weeks and will help to confirm clinical suspicions. Also, because CT and MRI stay normal in some patients, the SPECT changes may be the only imaging confirmation of brain dysfunction.

FIGURE 1. Demonstrates a normal HMPAO SPECT with symmetrical perfusion throughout the brain.

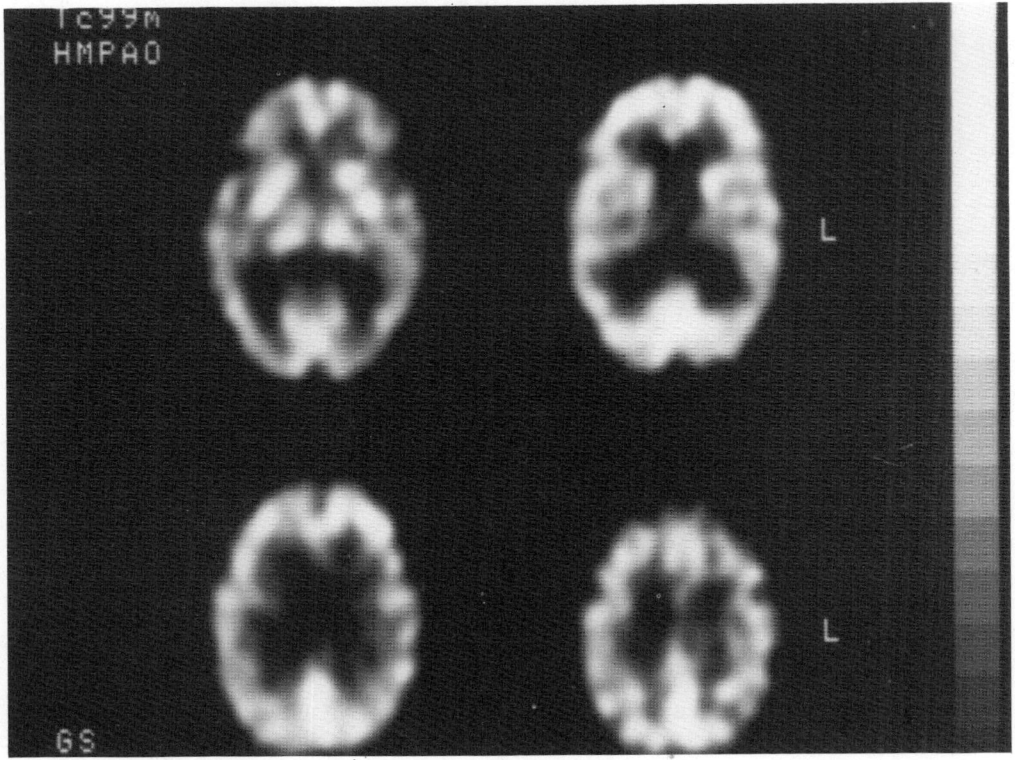

FIGURE 2. Demonstrates an HMPAO SPECT from a patient with a cocaine-induced left occipital stroke. There is a wedge-shaped area of hypoperfusion in the left occipital region, slight scalloped hypoperfusion in the periventricular regions and overall diminished cortical perfusion.

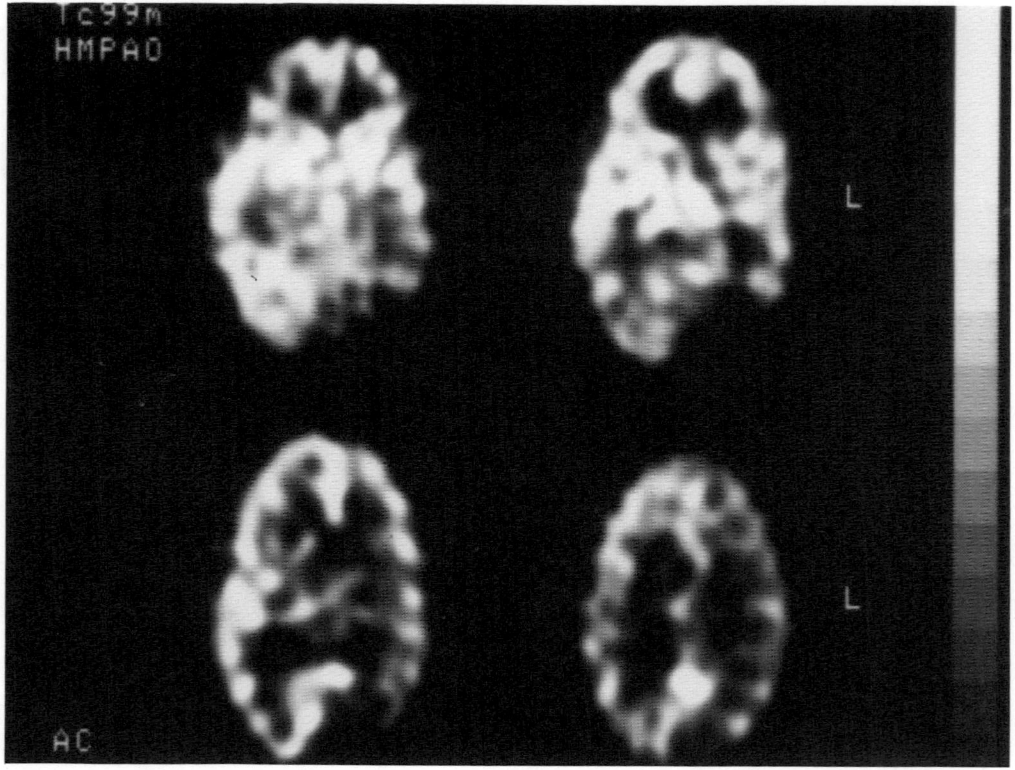

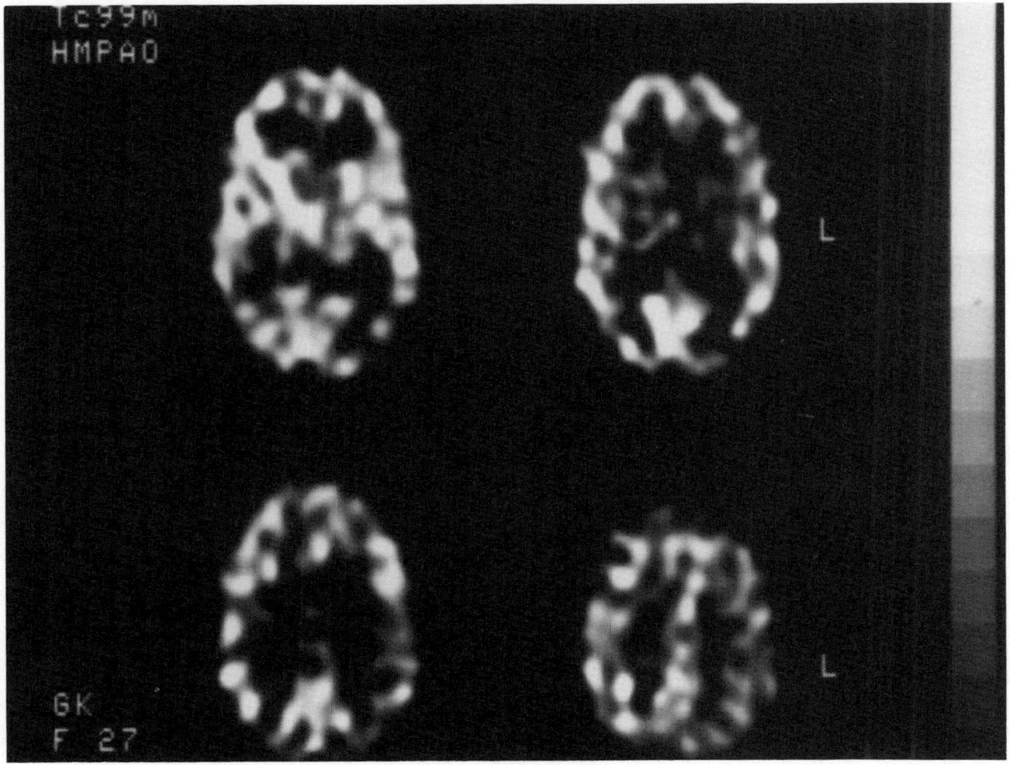

FIGURE 3. Is an HMPAO SPECT from a cocaine abuser with psychiatric symptoms. It demonstrates profound scalloping of perfusion to the periventricular regions. In addition, there are small multi-focal areas of cortical hypoperfusion. Overall cortical perfusion is profoundly diminished.

SPECT CHANGES WITH COCAINE ABUSE: PSYCHIATRIC COMPLICATIONS

We have started to evaluate patients with psychiatric complications from cocaine with SPECT. The majority of the patients studied have demonstrated manic or psychotic symptoms. In many there is a mixture of agitation, grandiosity, impaired judgement and psychosis. The patients with manic presentations resemble those with the "pseudopsychopathic personality disorder" described by Blumer and Benson in patients with orbito-frontal brain injury.[17] We have suspected that frontal lobe dysfunction occurs in association with the cocaine abuse even though structural studies of the brain such as CT or MRI have usually been normal. With SPECT we can test this hypothesis by measuring blood flow to the frontal regions.

The majority of the patients with "purely psychiatric" symptomatology had the same scalloping and multi-focal areas of hypoperfusion that was seen with SPECT in the neurologic patients. In addition, the patients with manic "pseudopsychopathic" syndromes have had selective hypoperfusion of the frontal lobes. These changes occurred in patients with normal CT and/or MRI suggesting that the SPECT is detecting abnormalities in function but not structure.

Previous work with positron emission tomography (PET) in patients with psychiatric symptoms associated with cocaine abuse showed decreased blood flow in the prefrontal regions.[18] One group proposed that the frontal hypoperfusion seen with PET may have been due to a depression that was associated with the cocaine abuse,[11] although, this hypothesis still needs further study.

Work with SPECT suggests that some of the psychiatric symptoms seen in cocaine abusers may have a vascular etiology. With other diseases that affect small blood vessels psychiatric symptoms can predominate. For example, the vasculitides including systemic lupus erythematosus can cause psychiatric symptomatology.[19] The cocaine-induced psychiatric symptoms may have a similar etiology. Further investigations of cocaine induced psychiatric symptoms may shed insight into patho-mechanisms for other psychiatric syndromes. Similarly, treatment strategies based on decreasing vasospasm should be considered in cocaine-induced psychiatric symptoms. Almost no work has been done in these areas.

CONCLUSIONS

Recent experience has demonstrated profound neurotoxicity associated with cocaine abuse. In many cases the toxicity is due to the spasm of cerebral blood vessels induced by excessive release of catecholamines. Stroke is a common consequence of this cocaine abuse. Psychiatric symptoms are also common and include mania, psychosis and depression.

SPECT appears to be a promising technology for assessing the effects of cocaine on brain function. It can demonstrate focal and multi-focal areas of hypoperfusion that explain clinical symptomatology when other imaging modalities are normal. One exciting direction for this work is further study of the hypothesis that some of the psychiatric syndromes seen with cocaine are due to cerebral ischemia. Further work quantitating and correlating cerebral blood flow with clinical symptoms is needed.

REFERENCES

1. National Institute on Drug Abuse *NIDA Notes* 1991; 5 (5): 11-14.

2. Gawin FH, Ellinwood, EN. Cocaine and other stimulants *New Engl. J. Med.* 1988; 318: 1173-1182.

3. Cregler, LL, Mark, H. Cardiovascular dangers of cocaine abuse. *Am. J. Card.* 1986; 57: 1185-1186.

4. Galloway, MP. Neurochemical interactions of cocaine with dopaminergic systems *Trends. Pharm. Sc.* 1988; 9: 452-454.

5. Volkow, ND, Wolf, AP., Dewey, S et al. Measurements of post synaptic dopamine receptors in cocaine abusers. *J. Nuc. Med.* 1989; 30: 730.

6. Rowley, HA, Lowenstein, DH, Rowbotham, MC, Simon, RP. Thalamomesencephalic strokes after cocaine abuse. *Neurology* 1989; 39: 428-430.

7. Mody, CK, Miller, BL, McIntyre, HB, Goldberg, MA. Neurological complications of cocaine abuse. *Neurology* 1988; 38: 1189-1193.

8. Levine, SR, Welch, KMA. Cocaine and stroke. *Stroke* 1988; 19:779-783.

9. Catravas JD, Waters, IW. Acute cocaine intoxication in the conscious dog: Studies on the mechanisms of lethality. *J Pharm Exp Ther* 1981; 217: 350-356.

10. Root, RK, Rowbotham, M. Neurologic aspects of cocaine abuse. *West J Med* 1988; 149: 442-448.

11. Baxter LR, Schwartz JM, Phelps ME et al. Localization of neurochemical effects of cocaine and other stimulants in the human brain. *J Clin Psychiatry* 1988;49 (suppl 2):23-26.

12. Jacobs IG, Roszler MH, Kelly JK et al. Cocaine abuse: Neurovascular complications. *Radiology* 1989;170:223-227.

13. Krendel DA, Ditter SM, Frankel MR, Ross WK. Biopsy-proven cerebral vasculitis associated with cocaine abuse. *Neurology* 1990;40:1092-1094.

14. Neirinckx RD, Canning LR, Piper IM et al. Technetium-99m d,1 HMPAO: A new radiopharmaceutical for SPECT imaging of regional cerebral perfusion. *J Nuc Med* 1987;28:191-202.

15. Miller BL, Garrett K, Leedom L et al. Neurospect in Cocaine Abuse: rCBF and HMPAO Findings. *Clin Nuc Med* 1989;14:12.

16. Mena I, Giombetti R, Mody CK et al. Acute cerebral blood flow changes with cocaine intoxication. *Neurology* (suppl 1) 1990 40;3:15.

17. Blumer D, Benson DF. Personality changes with frontal and temporal lobe lesion. In: Benson DF, Blumer D, eds. *Psychiatric aspects of neurological disease.* New York: Grune & Stratton, 1975:151-170.

18. Volkow ND, Mullani N, Gould KL et al. Cerebral blood flow in chronic cocaine user: a study with positron emission tomography. *Br J Psychiatry* 1988; 152:641-648.

19. Johnson RT, Richardson EP. The neurological manifestations of systemic lupus erythematosus. *Medicine* 1968;47:337.

Respiratory Effects of Cocaine Freebasing Among Habitual Cocaine Users

Donald P. Tashkin, MD
David Gorelick, MD, PhD
Maria-Elena Khalsa, MD
Michael Simmons
Potter Chang, PhD

SUMMARY. Smoking of alkaloidal cocaine ("crack") has become increasingly prevalent in our society. Recent evidence suggests that crack smoking can cause acute respiratory symptoms, abnormalities in lung function and, in some instances, severe, life-threatening acute lung injury. To evaluate further the relationship between frequent cocaine smoking and respiratory symptoms and lung dysfunction, we studied a sample of 177 heavy, habitual smokers of free-base cocaine (mean 6.6 gm/wk for an average of 27 months) with or without concomitant smoking of tobacco and/or marijuana. Results in this sample were compared with those in a control sample of 75 age-, sex- and race-matched nonsmokers of cocaine who did or did not also smoke tobacco and/or marijuana. After controlling for the use of other smoked substances, heavy, habitual cocaine smoking was associated with the following: (1) a high frequency of

---

Donald P. Tashkin is affiliated with the Department of Medicine; David Gorelick and Maria-Elena Khalsa are affiliated with the Department of Psychiatry; Michael Simmons is affiliated with the Department of Medicine; and Potter Chang is affiliated with the Department of Biostatistics, UCLA Schools of Medicine and Public Health, Los Angeles, CA and the West Los Angeles Veterans Affairs Medical Center, Brentwood Division, Los Angeles, CA.

Address reprint requests to: Donald P. Tashkin, MD, Department of Medicine, UCLA School of Medicine, Los Angeles, CA 90024-1690.

The research reported in this paper was supported by grant RO1 DA 03018 from the National Institute on Drug Abuse.

acute respiratory symptoms (cough, black sputum, chest pain) in temporal association with freebase use; (2) an obstructive ventilatory abnormality involving the large airways; and (3) a mild but significant impairment in the diffusing capacity of the lung. These findings suggest that heavy, habitual crack smoking produces (1) respiratory tract injury manifested by acute respiratory symptoms and evidence of chronic airflow obstruction in large airways, and (2) an abnormality in diffusion of gas at the alveolar-capillary level. The mechanism of the diffusion defect is unknown but could reflect damage to the alveolar-capillary membrane. Further study of the magnitude, persistence, reversibility, mechanism and clinical significance of the abnormality in diffusing capacity is needed.

The striking increase in the use of cocaine in the U.S. over the past decade[1] has been accompanied by a parallel rise in medical complications associated with cocaine use.[2,3] Within the past few years, snorting of cocaine hydrochloride has been largely replaced by smoking of the freebase form of cocaine as the preferred method of use. Freebase cocaine (''crack,'' ''rock''), obtained by alkaline extraction of the hydrochloride salt, is more suitable for smoking due to its greater volatility and resistance to thermal decomposition. When freebase cocaine is smoked, a large fraction escapes pyrolysis,[4] is inhaled and enters the blood stream via the extensive pulmonary circulation. The resultant intoxication is as rapid in onset and intense as that following intravenous administration, thus accounting for the popularity of freebase smoking. Because the lung is the principal organ exposed to the combustion products of smoked cocaine, pulmonary complications would be expected to be prominent among the health consequences of this form of drug abuse. While much remains to be learned concerning the respiratory effects of cocaine freebasing, evidence is emerging implicating ''crack'' cocaine as a cause of respiratory dysfunction and disease. This presentation will review our current state of knowledge concerning the respiratory complications of smoking alkaloidal cocaine.

A number of respiratory symptoms have been reported in temporal association with the smoking of cocaine, including cough, production of black sputum, hemoptysis, chest pain, wheeze and shortness of breath.[5-8] The cough experienced after cocaine smoking is likely to be due to a neurogenic reflex from stimulation of subepithelial irritant receptors by noxious ingredients within the inhaled smoke. The black sputum could represent carbonaceous residue from the fuel used to ignite the cocaine (butane, alcohol-soaked cotton wads, matches). The mechanism of the hemoptysis is not clear, nor is the site of the bleeding in the respiratory tract. The mechanism of the chest pain is also unknown; it may represent a local sensory response to acute airway irritation by high concentrations of cocaine or other components within the smoke. Until now, the actual frequency of acute respiratory symptoms experienced in relation to cocaine smoking has not been systematically evaluated.

Pneumothorax and/or pneumomediastinum, manifested clinically by pleuritic chest pain with or without shortness of breath, have been reported in several patients after cocaine use.[9-12] These complications are most likely due to the common practice of deeply inhaling the cocaine vapor into the lung, followed by extended Valsalva maneuvers which increase intra-thoracic pressure. As a result, alveolar air is more likely to rupture into the pulmonary interstitium with dissection along the vessels and bronchi to the mediastinum or free pleural space. Similar complications have been noted in marijuana smokers who use a comparable smoking technique.[13-14]

Several cases of acute diffuse lung damage have recently been reported in temporal relation to cocaine smoking.[15-18] Cucco et al.[15] described a patient who developed acute non-cardiogenic pulmonary edema alter smoking freebase cocaine which resolved spontaneously within 72 hours. No obvious cause of the pulmonary edema other than cocaine inhalation was clinically apparent. The authors hypothesized that the smoked cocaine caused acute toxic lung injury with increased alveolar endothelial and epithelial permeability resulting in pulmonary edema. However, they could not exclude an additional component of neurogenic pulmonary edema due to sympathetically mediated intense pulmonary vasoconstriction causing a high-pressure fluid leak.

Patel et al.[16] reported a case of biopsy-proven bronchiolitis obliterans with organizing pneumonia in a patient who admitted to intense use of freebase cocaine before the onset of respiratory symptoms. The patient presented with fever, cough, shortness of breath and nodular opacities on chest X-ray. He rapidly developed severe, life-threatening hypoxemia which required intubation and mechanical ventilatory support but subsequently responded to corticosteroid therapy. The absence of identifiable infectious causes or other inhalational exposures led the authors to speculate that the lung injury in this freebase user was due to toxins produced by the combustion of cocaine or unknown contaminants in the freebase preparation.

Kissner and coworkers[17] described a daily crack smoker who, over a period of several months, developed three separate episodes of fever, cough and bronchospasm associated with pruritus, eosinophilia, elevated immunoglobulin E blood level and transient pulmonary infiltrates. Each episode followed a bout of prolonged and intense freebasing and resolved with abstinence from cocaine use, suggesting an allergic mechanism.

Murray and associates[18] reported a smoker of alkaloidal cocaine who developed life-threatening diffuse alveolar hemorrhage after repeated freebasing over a 2-week period. The patient presented with fever, shortness of breath, blood-streaked sputum and diffuse alveolar infiltrates on chest X-ray. Open lung biopsy revealed diffuse alveolar hemorrhage without evidence of vasculitis. Treatment with high concentrations of inspired oxygen were required. Spontaneous resolution ensued with abstinence from cocaine.

The mechanism of the cocaine-related lung injury apparent in the above cases is unknown but, as Ettinger[19] has suggested, could include the following: (1) cocaine-induced pulmonary vasoconstriction leading to anoxic cell damage; (2) a direct toxic effect of cocaine on the alveolar capillary endothelium; or (3) a hypersensitivity reaction to components in the freebase smoke.

Another reported respiratory complication of cocaine smoking is severe thermal injury to the conducting airways due to ignition of ether used in the freebasing process leading to severe tracheal stenosis requiring tracheal reconstructive surgery. In addition, provocation of severe bronchospasm has been reported in a few patients with underlying asthma after freebasing,[20] presumably due to nonspecific irritation of the airways by noxious components within the smoke.

These accounts of clinically striking pulmonary effects attributed to crack use are anecdotal. While indicative of the potential for freebasing to produce lung injury, these individual case reports provide no indication of the true frequency with which smoked cocaine might produce less obvious lung damage that could lead to more chronic and persistent pulmonary abnormalities, especially in continuing freebase smokers. In this regard, at least two previous studies have assessed the lung function of cocaine-dependent patients to ascertain whether habitual smoking of cocaine might cause functional pulmonary abnormalities at a time when respiratory symptoms and/or abnormal auscultatory findings may or may not be evident. In two patients hospitalized for cocaine abuse, Weiss et al.[21] found a mild impairment in the single-breath diffusing capacity of the lung for carbon monoxide (D_LCO), while chronic respiratory symptoms, abnormal physical findings and chest radiographic abnormalities were all absent. Itkonen and associates[5] studied 19 freebase smokers hospitalized for treatment of drug abuse. Most of these patients complained of cough and/or sputum production, but the physical examination and chest X-ray were both normal. Lung function measured at least several days after cocaine was last used revealed normal spirometry and lung volumes but a definitely abnormal D_LCO ($\leq$ 70% of predicted) in 10 of the 19 patients; mean D_LCO was 59% of predicted in these 10 patients. In the two subjects who were retested 7-14 months alter ceasing cocaine use, the abnormality in D_LCO persisted. On the other hand, submaximal exercise tests in all five subjects with an abnormal D_LCO who were tested revealed normal gas exchange, suggesting that the degree of diffusion impairment present at the time was not yet clinically significant.

The above findings are potentially important since a reduced D_LCO could reflect damage to the integrity of the alveolar epithelial-capillary endothelial interface. Therefore, the finding of a diffusion defect in a large fraction of asymptomatic heavy cocaine smokers suggests a high frequency of subclinical lung damage involving the critically important gas-exchanging surface of the lung. On the other hand, one of the patients of Weiss et al.[21] had a history of intravenous drug abuse and septic pulmonary emboli which could have accounted for the diffusion impairment, and the other patient smoked tobacco which could have contributed to the reduced D_LCO.[22] Moreover, the significance of the findings of Itkonen and coworkers can be criticized because of (1) their small sample size, which may not be representative of cocaine smokers in general, (2) the potentially confounding influence of other drug use, including tobacco, which was smoked by the majority of their patients, and (3) the absence of a control sample. A larger-scale study of possible respiratory complications of habitual cocaine smoking which attempts to control for the potentially confounding influence of other drug use and hazardous exposures is required. To address this need, the present study was conducted to evaluate the respiratory status of a large sample of habitual smokers of alkaloidal cocaine alone and in combination with other smoked substances who denied intravenous drug abuse. A comparison sample of age-, sex- and race-matched non-users of cocaine who did or did not smoke tobacco and/or marijuana was also studied.

Entry criteria for cocaine smokers ("cases") to be included in the study included age 21-50 years and a history of current or recent smoking of $\geq$ 0.1 gram/day (average) of cocaine and $\geq$ 1 year of use. Exclusionary criteria included the following: intravenous drug abuse (> 5 times/lifetime); smoking (> 20 times/lifetime) of other illicit substances (PCP, heroin, opium, methamphetamine) except for cannabis; a history of chronic lung disease (e.g., asthma, tuberculosis, interstitial lung disease, chest wall abnormality or recent pneumonia); and significant occupational exposure to hazardous dusts or fumes. The comparison sample ("controls") fulfilled the same entry criteria except for the requirement that they never smoked cocaine. Cocaine-smoking cases were recruited from among patients admitted to the West Los Angeles Veterans Affairs (VA) Medical Center inpatient drug treatment program, as well as participants in non-VA outpatient chemical dependency programs. Control subjects were recruited from among the employees at the West Los Angeles VA Medical Center and UCLA Hospital. A total of 177 cases who fulfilled all entry criteria were recruited. Eighty-three percent of the cases were Black, 9% Caucasian, 6.7% Hispanic and 1.1% Native American. Because of the preponderance of Black cases and the well-known influence of race on lung function,[23-25] an attempt was made to recruit mostly Black controls. Ninety-six percent of the 75 qualifying control subjects were Black, 3% Caucasian and 1.3% of other racial origin. Nine of the cases and 3 of the controls were female. Analyses of lung function results were confined to Black male participants, while respiratory symptoms were analyzed across all subjects.

All subjects underwent the following examination procedures: (1) a screening questionnaire (to determine eligibility for the study); (2) a detailed respiratory and drug use questionnaire modified from the ATS-DLD respiratory questionnaire[26] and the NIDA National Survey on Drug Abuse,[27] with the addition of 25 questions relating to the chronology, frequency, intensity and patterns of cocaine use, the methods of preparing, igniting and smoking the alkaloidal cocaine, and any acute respiratory symptoms experienced in temporal relation to smoking cocaine: (3) a physical examination; (4) chest X-rays (in selected subjects); and (5) a battery of pulmonary function tests. The latter included whole-body plethysmographic measurements of airway resistance and thoracic gas volume at functional residual capacity (FRC), timed spirometry, maximal expiratory flow-volume curves breathing air and a low-density (80% helium, 20% oxygen) gas mixture. single-breath nitrogen washout, subdivisions of lung volume by helium dilution, and single-breath diffusing capacity for carbon monoxide (D_LCO).

Of the cases and controls, 85% and 83%, respectively, were never or former smokers of marijuana, while 66% and 47%, respectively, were current tobacco smokers. On the average, the cases were slightly older than the controls (mean ages 36.2 and 32.1 years, respectively). Mean daily tobacco use of tobacco-smoking cases and controls was similar (14.8 and 14.2 cigarettes/day, respectively), as was cumulative lifetime tobacco use (13.2 and 10.7 pack-years, respectively). Cocaine use among the cases averaged 6.6 gm/wk for 27 months; mean cocaine use was roughly comparable across tobacco- and marijuana-smoking categories, except for a somewhat higher, but more variable, mean weekly use among the never-marijuana, non-tobacco smoking cases. The interval between the time of testing and the time when cocaine was last smoked by the cases varied between 1 and 180 days (mean 18 days); over 75% of the cases had last smoked cocaine within 1 month of testing and over 90% within 3 months of testing. Eighty-five percent of the cases smoked dealer-prepared cocaine freebase (''crack''), while the remainder prepared their own freebase. The vast majority of the cases used a glass pipe for smoking, while approximately one-half used a butane lighter and one-third a dipstick soaked in rum or alcohol to ignite the cocaine.

The prevalence of *acute* cardiorespiratory symptoms in temporal relation to cocaine smoking among the 164 cases is shown in Figure 1. Slightly over 45% of the cases coughed up black sputum on at least some occasions within 12 hours after smoking cocaine. Only a small proportion of the cases (6.1%) reported hemoptysis alter freebasing. A large fraction of the cases (40.9%) experienced chest pain within 1 hour of smoking crack; in over 60% of these cases the chest pain was aggravated by taking a deep breath. Cardiac palpitations within 1 hour of freebasing were experienced by over one-half of the cocaine smokers and are consistent with the well-known pharmacologic effects of cocaine[2] in which norepinephrine re-uptake by adrenergic nerve endings is blocked leading to excessive catecholamine exposure. None of the above symptoms was related to the method of igniting the cocaine, i.e., with a butane lighter versus a dipstick soaked in rum or alcohol.

Chronic respiratory symptoms that were evaluated included the following: cough or sputum production on most days for at least 3 months out of the year for 2 or more consecutive years; more than one episode of increased cough and sputum lasting 3 weeks or more within the last 3 years; wheezing on 20 or more days a year or associated with breathlessness; and shortness of breath with ordinary activity on ≥ 20 days a year. Chi square or Fisher's exact test[28] was used to compare the prevalence of chronic respiratory symptoms between cases and controls in the same marijuana and/or tobacco smoking category. In contrast to the large proportion of habitual "crack" users who complained of *acute* respiratory symptoms in temporal proximity to smoking cocaine, the prevalence of *chronic* respiratory symptoms in habitual cocaine smokers was not significantly different from that in control subjects in the same marijuana and/or tobacco smoking category, including the never-marijuana, non-tobacco smoking participants. Our failure to detect an association between habitual crack use and *chronic* respiratory symptoms contrasts with previous evidence of an abnormally high prevalence of chronic respiratory symptoms among habitual smokers of marijuana and/or tobacco.[29] The disparity between these find-

FIGURE 1. Percentage of 164 cocaine smoking subjects who reported acute cardiorespiratory symptoms (cough productive of black sputum, bloody sputum, chest pain and palpitations) in temporal relation to cocaine smoking. The occurrence of symptoms was not related to the subjects' method of igniting cocaine, i.e., with a butane lighter versus a dipstick soaked in rum or alcohol.

*Chest pain was worse with deep breath in 63% (within 1 hr) and in 66% (at other times).

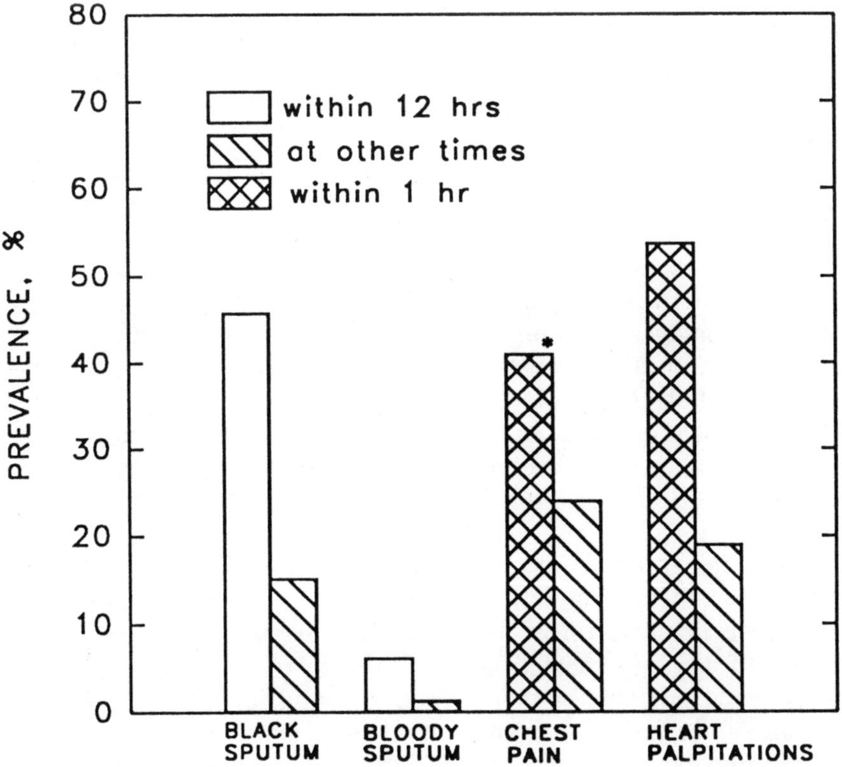

ings could be due to several factors. First, since our cocaine smokers had a relatively short total duration of habitual crack smoking (< 4 years), sufficient time may not have elapsed for these smokers to develop persistent respiratory symptoms for ≥ 2 years. Secondly, the cumulative lifetime quantity of cocaine smoked by our cases was relatively small in relation to the average daily amount of tobacco and/or marijuana smoked by those subjects who regularly used these substances. Thirdly, the histopathologic changes in the airways caused by the combustion products of cocaine may differ from the goblet cell metaplasia, loss of ciliated epithelium and inflammatory changes produced by chronic exposure to the smoke of tobacco or marijuana,[30] which share many of the same noxious components.[31,32]

Prevalence of lung function abnormality in the cocaine smokers was also compared with that in control subjects in the same tobacco and/or marijuana smoking category using contingency table analysis. Significant differences were noted only in never-marijuana, non-tobacco smoking participants, among whom the cases had a significantly higher frequency of abnormality in both D_LCO and in specific airway conductance (SG_{aw}) ($p < 0.05$). Our observation of significantly impaired diffusion in heavy, habitual cocaine smokers extends similar findings by Weiss et al.[21] and Itkonen and associates[5] in smaller numbers of patients. Moreover, these observations provide further support to the possibility that habitual exposure to smoked cocaine damages the pulmonary capillary membrane. Furthermore, our finding of an abnormally low specific airway conductance (an indicator of obstruction in large airways) in crack users suggests that habitual cocaine inhalation may injure the upper airway or the large intrathoracic bronchi, leading to airway narrowing. We have previously noted similar findings in heavy, habitual smokers of marijuana but not of tobacco.[29]

The clinical implications of the abnormality in diffusing capacity noted by others[5,21] and ourselves in heavy, habitual smokers of cocaine is unclear. Since the defect in diffusion was relatively mild, it would not be expected at this point to interfere with physical activity, as indicated by the absence of complaints of breathlessness by our subjects and the normal submaximal exercise tests performed by the patients of Itkonen et al.[5] On the other hand, the persistence of the diffusion abnormality weeks to months alter cessation of cocaine use and the possible relation of this physiologic abnormality to structural damage to the alveolar-capillary membrane suggest the possibility of progressive lung damage with continued use that could ultimately cause symptomatic impairment. Long-term follow-up studies of habitual crack users are needed to evaluate this possibility.

REFERENCES

1. National Survey Results. Johnston LD, O'Malley PM, Bachman JG. Drug use, drinking and smoking: National survey results from high schools, colleges, and young adults populations, 1975-1988. Natl Inst on Drug Abuse, USDHHS, Rockville, MD, DHHS Publ. No. (ADM) 89-1638,1989 (Public Health Service; Alcohol, Drug Abuse, and Mental Health Administration).

2. Cregler LL, Mark H. (Special Report) Medical complications of cocaine abuse. *N Engl J Med.* 1986; 315:1495-1500.

3. Bates CK. Medical risks of cocaine abuse (Specialty Conference). West J Med. 1988; 148:440-4.

4. Jeffcoat AR, Perez-Reyes M, Hill JM, Sadler BM, Cook CE. Cocaine disposition in humans alter intravenous injection, nasal insufflation (snorting), or smoking. *Drug Metab and Disposition.* 1989; 17:153-9.

5. Itkonen J, Schnoll S, Glassroth J. Pulmonary dysfunction in "freebase" cocaine users. *Arch Intern Med.* 1984; 144:2195-7.

6. Tashkin DP, Simmons MS, Coulson AH, Clark VA, Gong H Jr. Respiratory effects of cocaine "freebasing" among habitual users of marijuana with or without tobacco. *Chest.* 1987; 92:638-44.

7. Del Bono EA, O'Brien K, Murphy RLH Jr. Lung sound abnormalities in cocaine freebasers. *Substance Abuse.* 1989; 10:201-8.

8. Siegel RK Cocaine smoking. *J Psychoactive Drugs.* 1982; 14:277-359.

9. Shesser R, Davis C, Edelstein S. Pneumomediastinum and pneumothorax alter inhaling alkaloidal cocaine. *Ann Emerg Med.* 1981; 10:213-5.

10. Morris JB, Shuck JM. Pneumomediastinum in a young male cocaine user. *Ann Emerg Med.* 1985; 14:194-6.

11. Bush MN, Rubenstein R, Hoffman I, Bruno MS. Spontaneous pneumomediastinum as a consequence of cocaine use (Case Report). *NY State J Med.* 1984; 84:618-9.

12. Aroesty DJ, Stanley RB Jr, Crockett DM. Pneumomediastinum and cervical emphysema from the inhalation of "free based" cocaine. Report of three cases. *Otolaryngeal Head Neck Surg.* 1986; 94:372-4.

13. Miller WE, Spiekerman BE, Hepper NG. Pneumomediastinum resulting from performing Valsalva maneuvers during marijuana smoking. *Chest.* 1972; 62:233-4.

14. Mattox KL. Pneumomediastinum in heroin and marijuana users. *JACEP.* 1976; 5:26-8.

15. Cucco RA, Yoo OH, Cregler L, Chang JC. Nonfatal pulmonary edema alter "freebase" cocaine smoking. *Am Rev Resp Dis.* 1987; 136:179-81.

16. Patel RC, Dutta D, Schonfeld SA. Free-base cocaine use associated with bronchiolitis obliterans organizing pneumonia. *Ann Intern Med.* 1987; 107:186-7.

17. Kissner DG, Lawence WD, Sells JE, Flint A. Crack lung: Pulmonary disease caused by cocaine abuse. *Am Rev Respir Dis.* 1987; 136:1250-2.

18. Murray RJ, Albin RJ, Mergner W, Criner GJ. Diffuse alveolar hemorrhage temporally related to cocaine smoking. *Chest.* 1988; 93:427-9.

19. Ettinger NA, Albin RJ. A review of the respiratory effects of smoking cocaine. *Am J Med.* 1989; 87:664-8.

20. Rebhun J. Associations of asthma and freebase smoking. *Ann Allergy.* 1988; 60:339-42.

21. Weiss RD, Goldenheim PD, Mirin SM, Hales CA, Mendelson JH. Pulmonary dysfunction in cocaine smokers. *Am J Psychiatry.* 1981; 138:1110-2.

22. Martt JM. Pulmonary diffusing capacity in cigarette smokers. *Ann Intern Med.* 1962; 56:39-45.

23. Seltzer CC, Siegelaub AB, Friedman GD, Collen MF. Differences in pulmonary function related to smoking habits and race. *Am Rev Respir Dis.* 1974; 110:598-608.

24. Lanese RR, Keller MD, Foley MF, Underwood EH. Differences in pulmonary function tests among whites, blacks, and American Indians in a textile company. *JOM.* 1978; 20:39-44.

25. Schoenberg JB, Beck GJ, Bouhuys A. Growth and decay of pulmonary function in healthy blacks and whites. *Respir Physiology.* 1978; 33:367-93.

26. Ferris BG. Epidemiology Standardization Project. *Am Rev Respir Dis.* 1978; 118/6(Part 2): 1-88.

27. Fishburne PM, Abelson HI, Cisin I. National Survey on Drug Abuse: Main Findings, 1979. Rockville, MD. Natl Inst on Drug Abuse 1980. DHHS Publication No (ADM) 80-976.

28. Siegel S. Nonparametric statistics for the behavioral sciences. New York: McGraw Hill, 1956.

29. Tashkin DP, Coulson AH, Clark VA et al. Respiratory symptoms and lung function in habitual heavy smokers of marijuana alone, smokers of marijuana and tobacco, smokers of tobacco alone, and nonsmokers. *Am Rev Respir Dis.* 1987; 135:209-16.

30. Fligiel SEG, Beals TF, Venkat H, Stuth S, Gong H, Tashkin DP. Pulmonary pathology in marijuana smokers. In: Marijuana–An International Research Report. *Proceedings of the Melbourne Symposium on Cannabis*, Sept. 1987. Monograph Series No. 7. Chesher G, Consroe P, Musty R, eds. Canberra, Australian Government Publishing Service, 1988, pp. 43-8.

31. Hoffman D, Brunneman DK, Gori GB et al. On the carcinogenicity of marijuana smoke. *Recent Adv Phytochem* 1975; 9:63-81.

32. Novotný M, Merli F, Weisler D et al. Fractionation and capillary gas chromatographic-mass spectrometric characterization of the neutral components in marijuana and tobacco smoke condensates. *J Chromatogr.* 1982; 238:140-50.

Cardiovascular Effects and Toxicities of Cocaine

Koonlawee Nademanee, MD

SUMMARY. Cocaine exerts a myriad of adverse cardiovascular effects which are dependent on the dose, rate of administration, and duration of use. The drug has two primary pharmacologic actions: it is a powerful sympathomimetic agent and a local anesthetic. The drug blocks the presynaptic reuptake of catecholamines resulting in the marked hormonal increase at the postsynaptic receptor sites. These effects, in turn, lower the threshold for coronary vasoconstriction and vasospasm, myocardial ischemia and infarction. In addition, the drug's multiple pharmacologic and electrophysiologic cardiovascular actions can promote arrhythmias, myocarditis, cardiomyopathy, as well as unmasking subclinical diseases. Long-term cocaine use can cause autonomic disturbances and alter catecholamine homeostasis: chronic cocaine addicts face serious cardiovascular sequelae from the drug's multiple adverse effects. It is important to assess the prevalence of cocaine-related cardiovascular diseases, to understand how the drug affects the autonomic nervous system, and to determine its long-term effects on the cardiovascular system.

INTRODUCTION

Cocaine use rose swiftly in the 1980s when the drug became available in freebase form, which generally is cheaper, purer, and faster acting than cocaine hydrochloride.[1] As more people used the

---

Koonlawee Nademanee is Professor of Medicine, University of Colorado and Chief of Cardiology, Denver General Hospital, 660 Bannock Street, Denver, CO 80204.

Address reprint requests to: Dr. Koonlawee Nademanee, at Denver General Hospital, 660 Bannock Street, Denver, CO 80204.

The research reported in this paper was supported in part by grant #R01 DA04 585-03 from the National Institute on Drug Abuse, Rockville, MD, and in part by the American Heart Association. (Grant-in Aid) #789 GI-3.

drug, more reports of various cocaine-related cardiovascular complications were published.[2-4] This is not surprising: cocaine has many deleterious pharmacological effects on the cardiovascular system even in people who are not otherwise at risk for coronary artery disease (e.g., premenopausal women, young, otherwise healthy athletes, men with no associated risk factors).[4] We have been seeing in emergency rooms and coronary care units patients who have symptoms' of heart disease that had until now been restricted to high risk populations. And although current statistics show that fewer people are using cocaine, many addicts continue to use the drug. For these reasons, research investigating cocaine-related cardiovascular disease should continue.

Cocaine Pharmacokinetics and Metabolism

Cocaine is derived from *Erythroxylon coca* leaves.[5] The drug is an alkaloid which when dissolved in hydrochloric acid forms cocaine hydrochloride, a water-soluble salt. Cocaine follows the two-compartment model:[6,7] it has a steady-state volume of distribution averaging 132 L or 1.96 L/kg. Its elimination clearance is 2.10 L/min and the elimination phase half-life is 48 minutes. Its chronotropic effect peaks 7.3 minutes after an intravenous dose.[6] Biophase cocaine concentrations initially increase heart rate by 0.3 bpm for each 1 ng/ml.[7] The chronotropic effects of intravenous cocaine decline more rapidly than plasma levels or biophase concentrations.

Plasma and liver cholinesterase detoxify cocaine into two water-soluble metabolites, benzoylecgonine and ecgonine methyl ester.[6] Both metabolites are excreted in the urine, and traces of these metabolites may be found in the urine up to 36 hours after ingestion, depending on how the drug was taken or the rate of cholinesterase activity. Because pregnant women, fetuses, infants, elderly men and patients who have liver disease or a congenital cholinesterase deficiency have diminished cholinesterase function, they are more sensitive to cocaine than healthy adults.

The Effects of Cocaine on Neurotransmitters and Autonomic Function

Cocaine blocks the presynaptic reuptake of catecholamines, more of which become available at the post-synaptic receptor sites.[8] The drug also sensitizes peripheral organs and central nervous system to the effects of circulating catecholamines, inhibits monoamine oxidase, and exerts direct anti-cholinergic effects.[9] Taken together, these acute effects could increase sympathetic activity resulting in increased heart rate, blood pressure and vasoconstriction.[10]

When the drug is used chronically, the mechanisms governing cocaine-induced cardiovascular and neurochemical disorders are more complex. The receptors develop a tolerance to dopamine and norepinephrine.[11] The resultant increase in sympathetic activity or α-response to stimulation is much less than when the drug is used the first time.[12] Also, after repeated use of cocaine, any increase in the concentration of neurotransmitters may not be as significant as when the drug is used the first time. So when a chronic cocaine user withdraws from the drug, the postsynaptic receptors could be supersensitive to sympathetic stimulation–either direct or behavioral.

The nature of cocaine addiction is such that the addicts use the drug irregularly, typically in binges and then stopping for several days. This means that cocaine-induced cardiovascular disturbances and neurochemical imbalances are dynamic. An addict's risk of developing myocardial ischemia or infarct may not be as great during the binge itself as afterward during withdrawal. During the binge, changes in blood pressure, heart rate, and vasoconstriction may not be significant because a tolerance may have developed. But when the addict withdraws from the drug, supersensitivity of the adrenergic receptors to external stimuli may be heightened, and he would then be more prone to develop cardiovascular complications. This is why it is simplistic to speculate that the acute effects of the drug in cocaine addicts are the primary and sole causal factor for cardiovascular complications (e.g., ischemia, infarct).

CARDIOVASCULAR EFFECTS

Systemic and Coronary Hemodynamics

Cocaine has profound effects on the coronary vasculature. The drug stimulates the α-receptors, causing coronary and systemic vasoconstriction.[13-15] Lange et al. demonstrated that intranasal doses of cocaine HCL as small as 10% (2 mg per kilogram of body-weight) decreased the coronary diameter by 8-12% and coronary sinus blood flow by 17%.[12] Even at doses within the range of topical anesthesia, cocaine increased myocardial oxygen demand while causing vasoconstriction. Because these effects can be reversed by phentolamine, an α-blocking agent, investigators attribute them to stimulation of the α-adrenergic receptors.[12] This fits nicely with a subsequent report showing that ß-blockade worsens cocaine-induced vasoconstriction.

Cocaine also enhances the calcium influx across the cell membrane, which in turn augments vascular smooth muscle tone. This effect is independent of the drug's action in potentiating smooth muscle response to catecholamines.[4] However, these effects on the α-receptors and calcium influx could cause vasospasm. While there is no conclusive evidence supporting this theory, several reports cite vasospasm of infarct-related vessels as the cause of acute myocardia infarction in cocaine addicts.[2]

Effects on Myocardial Contractility

Considerable evidence suggests that cocaine has a negative inotropic effect on myocardial contractility. Fraker et al.[16] found that a 4 mg intravenous dose of cocaine administered to conscious dogs quickly depressed the regional ejection fraction as much as 50%; this effect dissipated within ten minutes. Comparable findings were observed in pentobarbital-sedated dogs; these sedated dogs did not exhibit a significant increase in heart rate and blood pressure which might have affected left ventricular function. Fraker et al. concluded that cocaine directly depresses myocardial function rather than influencing it indirectly through changes in oxygen demand. Hale et al.[17] and Abel et al.[18] concluded that the impaired left ventricular performance in anesthetized dogs was a function of cocaine's cumulative effects.

Electrophysiologic Effects

Like other local anesthetics, cocaine has Class I antiarrhythmic properties. Cocaine blocks the fast sodium channel, depresses cardiac depolarization and conduct ion, and extends the duration of QRS complex, QT interval and refractoriness of cardiac muscle.[19]

The electrophysiologic effects of cocaine are also modulated by sympathomimetic effects of the drug. In humans, a 48 mg dose of intravenous cocaine HCL increases the sinus rate and shortens the AV nodal refractory period and conduction; at this dose, cocaine has only a slight effect on the His-Purkinje conduction. There is no evidence suggesting that smaller doses of cocaine provoke life-threatening arrhythmias, unless the drug is given in patients who have an arrhythmia substrate (e.g., Wolfe-Parkinson-White syndrome, myocardial ischemia, or myocardial infarction). However, at larger ($>$ 50 mg doses), cocaine's sodium channel-blocking effects may become more evident, thereby increasing ventricular and His-Purkinje conduction time. This can precipitate arrhythmias such as ventricular tachycardia or bradyarrhythmia.

Acute Myocardial Infarction

The number of people using cocaine has increased and so has the incidence of acute MI temporally related to its use.[2-4] Acute myocardial infarction is the most frequently reported cardiac complication of cocaine use. Most patients are chronic cocaine users; however, in rare instances, a first-time user could suffer MI.[4] The argument that the rise in the number of cocaine users suffering acute myocardial infarction is strictly a function of the growing number of people using the drug is not compelling because most cases of cocaine-related acute myocardial infarction occurred in relatively young individuals (mean age 31 years) and at the same rate for males and females. Coronary angiography performed in cocaine-related infarct patients shows a high prevalence of normal coronary arteries (31%), and 35% had evidence of thrombogenic formation in the infarcted vessel.[20]

Both acute and chronic cocaine use may lower the thresholds for myocardial ischemia and myocardial infarction. A powerful sympathomimetic, cocaine provides a milieu for myocardial ischemia and infarction. Acute cocaine administration immediately increases heart rate, blood pressure, and myocardial oxygen demand, lowering the threshold for vasospasm. Acute cocaine administration may also cause vasoconstriction, particularly in patients who have preexisting coronary obstruction because the drug further impedes blood flow by increasing vascular resistance. As mentioned, cocaine also enhances platelet stickiness,[21] in turn promoting thrombus formation. When these effects coincide with increased oxygen demand, myocardial ischemia is more likely to ensue.

Chronic cocaine use can reduce dopamine levels at the synapses, thereby sensitizing the α-adrenergic receptors and lowering the threshold for vasospasm. There is evidence suggesting that cocaine addicts are more likely to develop vasospasm which may lead to acute myocardial infarction during the early stages of withdrawal from the drug. Zimmermann et al.[22] described a cocaine addict who had recurrent transient ST-elevation typical of vasospasm. The patient's first coronary angiogram was normal with a negative ergonovine-induced spasm. However, his symptoms and ST-elevation recurred during hospitalization when he was not using the drug. A second angiogram revealed a complete left anterior descending artery occlusion. This case suggests that habitual cocaine users face a continued risk of developing vasospasm and acute myocardial infarction even after they stop using the drug for several days.

Myocardial Ischemia in Cocaine Addicts

To determine the prevalence of myocardial ischemia in cocaine addicts, we studied 21 male patients (mean age 34 ± 6 years) who had used cocaine for at least six months prior to the study and enrollment in a 28-day inpatient treatment program.[23] The majority had used the drug in freebase form at an average dose of 1.8 g/day. The mean interval between the last use of cocaine and admission was nine days, and the mean duration of cocaine use was 27 months. Eight of the 21 patients enrolled in the study (38%) had a history of chest pain, but none had suffered a myocardial infarction.

After giving informed consent, the subjects underwent exercise treadmill testing and 24-hour Holter monitoring. All patients had their first Holter monitoring during the first two weeks after admission, and so the number of days from the last dose of cocaine and the first Holter varied considerably. Of the 21 initial Holter tapes, four could not be analyzed due to mechanical failure, early removal of electrodes by patens, or other reasons. Sixteen patients had a second Holter within three to four weeks after admission, five of whom had another Holter six to twelve weeks after admission. Abstinence from cocaine during the testing period was verified by urine assays. The Holter tapes were coded, scanned blindly and mixed with those of 119 angina patients (70 stable angina; 49 unstable angina) and 42 healthy volunteers (age 28.7 ± 3.6 years), none of whom had a history of heart disease or coronary risk factors.

We found that the cocaine addicts had ST elevation episodes during withdrawal (mean duration per episode: 57 ± 77 minutes; range: one to 362 minutes): 45% during the first week of withdrawal, 25% during the second, 28% during the third, and 11% during the fourth. No ischemic episodes occurred after six weeks of withdrawal. These ST changes resembled those of Prinzmetal angina patients (Figure 1).

A significantly greater proportion of cocaine addicts had ST elevation episodes than either the volunteer or angina patient groups. Eight of the 21 cocaine addict patients (38%) had a total of 45 ST elevation episodes (range: one to 13 episodes per 24-hour period; mean 5.6 episodes). In contrast, only 4% of the unstable angina patients had ST elevation episodes; one chronic stable angina patient had ST elevation episodes; no volunteers had these episodes. These findings suggest that cocaine users increase their risk of developing ST changes by a factor of 16 when compared with the volunteers, and that this risk continues even after they cease using the drug.

Only one of the 20 cocaine addicts tested positive for exercise-induced myocardial ischemia, indicating that most did not have significant coronary artery obstruction. Only three of the 42 volunteers had ST changes characteristic of myocardial ischemia during exercise treadmill testing.

Our findings support the theory that chronic cocaine use predisposes coronary arteries to vasospasm, an effect lingering well into withdrawal. This may be explained by the hypothesis that chronic cocaine use depletes the dopamine levels.[9,11] Dopamine, a powerful coronary vasodilator, stimulates the dopamine receptors in the coro-

FIGURE 1. St elevation episode on Holter monitoring in a patient with normal coronary arteries and negative ergonovine test. Panel A shows QRS complex with normal ST segment before the episode of ST elevation (Panel B). Panel C shows biphasic T waves immediately after ST elevation episode. Panel D shows normal ST segment during peak exercise. (Reprinted with permission from Ann Int Med 1989; 111:876-880; 12/1/89.)

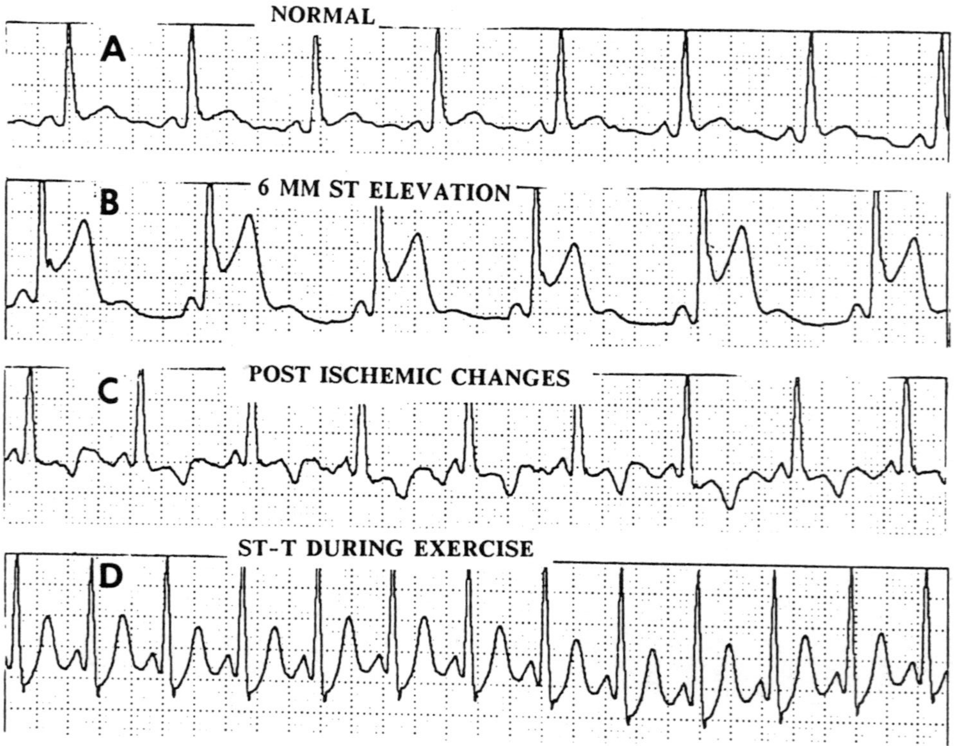

nary arteries and inhibits norepinephrine release at the presynaptic junction.[24] A lack of dopamine may lower the threshold for vasospasm and enhance the release norepinephrine. Several studies have shown that long-term use of stimulants causes the central dopaminergic α-adrenergic and ß-adrenergic receptors to become supersensitive. According to Gawin and Kleber,[25] the primary neurophysiologic substrate of cocaine withdrawal is a heightened sensitivity of the inhibitor receptors on the dopamine neuron (autoreceptors), which weakens dopaminergic transmission. By causing dopamine depletion, chronic cocaine use could sensitize the α-adrenergic receptors, lowering the threshold for vasospasm. The finding that cocaine users experience a marked rise in blood pressure in response to exercise immediately after withdrawal is consistent with this hypothesis.

Cardiac Arrhythmias and Sudden Cardiac Death

The multiple pharmacologic and electrophysiologic actions of cocaine can promote cardiac arrhythmias. Cocaine, by destabilizing the electrophysiologic properties of arrhythmogenic substrates or by provoking arrhythmogenic effects by sympathetic stimulation, precipitates arrhythmias ranging from bradyarrhythmia to ventricular fibrillation.[4,19] Patients who have accessory pathways, a prior myocardial infarction, or myocarditis are already prone to develop refractory arrhythmias. But they are even more prone to develop malignant arrhythmias–that may ultimately lead to sudden cardiac death–when they use cocaine.

Myocarditis, Cardiomyopathy, and Miscellaneous Cardiovascular Complications

Virmani et al.,[26] in their study of sudden traumatic death victims whose body fluids had detectable levels of cocaine in their body fluids, found evidence of myocarditis in 20% (eight of 40 patients); histologic examination of these hearts showed mononuclear infiltrate with prominent eosinophilic component. In contrast, only 3.7% (one in 27) of sudden traumatic death victims whose body fluids were free of cocaine showed evidence of myocarditis. The authors concluded that myocarditis occurred frequently in patients dying of cocaine abuse and may be a function of microvascular injury.

Two cases of cocaine-induced myocarditis progressing to dilated cardiomyopathy with congestive heart failure were reported by Wiener et al.[27] One patient had chest pain and elevated levels of cardiac enzymes; his coronary arteries were normal. The other patient (a 28-year old woman) presented with symptoms of biventricular failure and dilatation; her coronary arteries were also normal.

A case of reversible cardiomyopathy associated with cocaine intoxication was recently described by Chokshi et al.[28] A 35-year old woman had been smoking crack cocaine all day; she entered the hospital because of seizure, respiratory failure and severe congestive heart failure. The first echocardiogram showed left ventricular dilatation with severe global left ventricular hypokinesis (ejection fraction of 10%). There was no evidence of acute MI, and supportive therapy was successful. Another echocardiogram two weeks later showed a nondilated left ventricle (ejection fraction of 49%). This case of cocaine-induced cardiomyopathy mimics the catecholamine cardiomyopathy one sees in patients who have pheochromocytoma. Clearly, high levels of catecholamines circulating to the heart are very toxic–whether caused by an adrenal tumor or cocaine. High doses of cocaine can increase blood pressure to 250 HG or more which may cause cardiovascular complications of several subclinical diseases such as dissecting aneurysms, subarachnoid hemorrhage or rupture of the ascending aorta.

CONCLUSION

Cocaine exerts pharmacologic effects by means of powerful sympathomimetic and local anesthetic actions. The drug blocks the presynaptic uptake of catecholamines, thereby potentiating sympathetic responses. Acute and chronic cocaine administration could alter autonomic homeostasis; this in turn may provoke vasospasm and narrow the coronary and systemic vasculature. These cocaine-induced complications may occur even during withdrawal, and may trigger episodes of myocardial ischemia, acute myocardial infarction, and myocarditis. Cardiac arrhythmias and cardiomyopathy are associated with chronic cocaine use. Research is needed so that clinicians can better treat cocaine-induced heart disease.

REFERENCES

1. Jekel JF, Podlewski H, Dean-Patterson S, Allen DF, Clarke N, Cartwright P. Epidemic Free-base Cocaine Abuse. Lancet 1986;1459-62.

2. Isner JM, Estes NAM III, Thompson PD, Costanzo-Nordin MR, Subramanian R, Miller G, Katsas G, Sweeney K, and Sturner WQ. Acute cardiac events temporally related to cocaine use. N Eng J Med 1986;315:1438-43.

3. Cregler LL, Mark H. Medical complications of cocaine abuse. N Eng J Med 1986;315:1495-1500.

4. Isner, J.M, Chokshi S.K.: Cocaine-related Heart disease: In Heart Disease Update; edited by Braunwald E: 1991;323-333.

5. Freud S: Ueber coca. Centralblatt fur die gesamte Therapie 1884;2:289-3 14.

6. Stewart DJ, Inaba T, Lucassen M, Kalow W. Cocaine metabolism: Cocaine and norcocaine hydrolysis by liver and serum esterases. Clin Pharmacol Ther 1979;25:464-468.

7. Chow MJ, Ambre JJ, Ruo TI et al. Kinetics of cocaine distribution, elimination, and chronotropic effects. Clin Pharmacol Ther 1985;38:3 18-324.

8. Ritchie JM, Green NM: Local Anesthetics. In Gilman AG, Goodman LS, Rall TW, Murad F, eds. The pharmacologic basis of therapeutics 7th ed. New York: MacMillan 1985:309-10.

9. Kalivas PW, Duffy P, Du Mars, LA, Skinner, C. Behavioral and neurochemical effects of acute and daily cocaine administration in rats. J Pharmacol. Exp. Ther. 245:485-492, 1988.

10. Resnick RB, Kestenbaum RS, Schwartz LK. Acute systemic effects of cocaine in man: a controlled study by intranasal and intravenous routes. Science 1977 (Feb);195:696-8.

11. Avakian EV, Leroy M, St John-Allan K, Sayre FW, Malone, MH. Effects of chronic cocaine administration and cocaine withdrawal on coronary flow rate and heart rate responses to epinephrine and cocaine in isolated perfused rat hearts. Life Sciences; 46:1569-1574, 1990.

12. Javas JI, Fischman MW, Schuster CR, Dekirmenjian H, Davis JM. Cocaine plasma concentration: relation to physiological and subjective effects in humans. Science October 1978; 202:227-8.

13. Lange RA, Cigarroa RG, Yancy CW Jr. et al. Cocaine-induced coronary-artery vasoconstriction. N Engl J Med 1989;321:1557-1562.

14. Lange RA, Cigarroa RG, Eduardo D, McBride W, Kim AS, Wells PJ, Bedotto JB, Danziger RS, Hillis LD. Potentiation of cocaine-induced coronary vasoconstriction by beta-adrenergic Blockade. Ann Internal Med. 112:897-903; 1990.

15. Flores ED, Lange R., Cigarroa, Hillis LD: Effects of cocaine on coronary artery dimensions in atherosclerotic coronary artery disease: enhanced vasoconstriction at sites of significant stenosis. JACC. 16;74-79, 1990.

16. Fraker TD, Temesy-Armos PN, Brewster PS et al. Mechanism of cocaine-induced myocardial depression in dogs. Circulation 1990;81: 1012-1016.

17. Hale SL, Alker KJ, Rezkala S et al. Cardiodepressant effects of cocaine, abstracted. J Am Coll Cardiol 1989;13:78A.

18. Abel FL, Wilson SP, Zhao RR, Fennell WH: Cocaine depresses the canine myocardium. Circulatory Shock 1989;28:309-319.

19. Temesy-Armos PN, Fraker TD, Wilkerson RW. Cardiac electrophysiological effects of cocaine in animal models. In NIDA Research Monograph Series. 108:131-138;1991.

20. Smith HW 3d, Liberman HA, Brody, Battey LL, Donahue BC, Morris DC. Acute myocardial infarction temporally related to cocaine use: clinical, angiographic, and pathophysiologic observation. Ann Intern Med 1987;107(1):13-8.

21. Kleinbaum D, Kupper L, Morgenstern H. Epidemiologic Research, New York: Van Nostrand Reinhold; 1982:297-99.

22. Zimmerman FH, Gustafson GM, Kemp HG Jr. Recurrent myocardial infarction associated with cocaine abuse in a young man with normal coronary arteries: evidence for coronary artery spasm culminating in thrombosis. J Am Coll Cardiol 1987; 91(Apr):964-8.

23. Nademanee K, Gorelick DA, Josephson MA et al. Myocardial ischemia during cocaine withdrawal. Ann Intern Med 1989;111:876-880.

24. Goldberg LI, Rajfer SI. Dopamine receptor: applications in clinical cardiology. Circulation 1985;72:245-8.

25. Gawin FH, and Kleber HD. Abstinence symptomatology and psychiatric diagnosis in cocaine abusers. Arch Gen Psychiatry 1986;43: 107-13.

26. Virmani R, Robinowitz M, Smialek JE, Smyth DF. Cardiovascular effects of cocaine: an autopsy study of 40 patients. Am Heart J 1988;115(5):1068-76.

27. Wiener RS, Lockhart JT, Schwartz RG. Dilated cardiomyopathy and cocaine abuse: Report of two cases. Am J Med 1986;81:699-701.

28. Chokshi SK, Moore R, Pandian NG, Isner JM. Reversible cardiomyopathy associated with cocaine intoxication. Ann Intern Med 1989;111:1039-1040.

Observations on Increased CPK Levels in "Asymptomatic" Cocaine Abusers

W. Garnet Warrian, MD
James A. Halikas, MD
Ross D. Crosby, PhD
Gregory A. Carlson, BS
Fred Crea, BS

SUMMARY. In order to assess increased creatinine phosphokinase (CPK) among medically asymptomatic active crack cocaine abusers, retrospective analysis of daily supervised urine data collected in a 20 day daily visit plus 12 week followup weekly visit study of heavy crack cocaine abusers was performed. The subjects were 36 black male chronic crack cocaine users unmotivated in drug abuse treatment, willing to be studied for daily payment, who were recruited by word of mouth on the street. Of the 464 CPK results obtained, the mean CPK value was 397 (SD = 784) IU/L. Two-thirds of the results were greater than 200; 19% were greater than 500 IU/L. CPK test results were systematically eliminated if related to medical causes or concurrent other drug use. The relative contribution of recent alcohol use versus recent cocaine use in raising CPK was assessed by dividing the remaining 435 observations into sequential

---

W. Garnet Warrian is a fourth year medical student, University of Manitoba, Faculty of Medicine. James A. Halikas is Professor of Psychiatry, University of Minnesota School of Medicine, and Director, Chemical Dependency Treatment Program, University of Minnesota Hospital and Clinic. Ross D. Crosby is a Biostatistician and Senior Research Scientist, Department of Psychiatry, University of Minnesota. Gregory A. Carlson is Administrative Director, Chemical Dependency Treatment Program, University of Minnesota. Fred Crea is Clinical Coordinator, Cocaine Treatment Program, Chemical Dependency Treatment Program, University of Minnesota.

Address correspondence and reprint requests to: James A Halikas, MD, Professor of Psychiatry, University of Minnesota, Box 393 UMHC, Minneapolis, MN 55455.

use groups. With alcohol use instances excluded, a statistically significant relationship between urine cocaine metabolite and elevated CPK was found. When all other possible causes of elevated CPK levels were controlled, crack cocaine use was associated with a significant quantitative effect on CPK level.

The recreational use of cocaine has dramatically increased in the past decade. Cocaine was reported to be the most commonly abused drug requiring emergency room visits in the United States as early as 1986.[1] The nearly pure form of cocaine, "crack," has come into alarmingly wide use due to its increasing availability and decreasing street price.[2,3,4] This smoked form of cocaine is effectively absorbed by the respiratory system and results in a rapid increase in plasma concentration.[5] Clinically, crack appears to be the most rapidly addicting form of cocaine devised. It has even been speculated that the "first time" user may be more susceptible to the potentially fatal effects of acute high plasma cocaine concentrations than the more tolerant habitual user.[6] A combination of increasing prevalence of cocaine abuse and a significantly more addicting method of administration make "crack use" a serious health threat.[7,8]

Descriptions of acute presentations of cocaine intoxication as well as cardiovascular and central nervous system effects of cocaine have been extensively reported.[7-11] A previously infrequently described, but clinically significant, complication of cocaine use is rhabdomyolysis (RML). Rhabdomyolysis, literally "lysis of the muscle cell," connotes a pathological process in which the integrity of the muscle cell is altered and the cellular components (e.g., enzymes) spill into the extracellular space. One of the enzymes released is creatinine phosphokinase (CPK). Its detection in the serum in elevated amounts is the basis upon which various algorithms are developed for making the diagnosis of RML. Recently there has been a dramatic increase in reported cases of cocaine-associated RML from emergency room settings.[3-5,12-26] Often these cases have been associated with acute renal failure (ARF).[27-28] To date, however, no reports of incidentally identified RML in "asymptomatic" outpatient cocaine abusers have been cited.

METHODOLOGY

Data from an outpatient study of 32 chronic crack cocaine users was retrospectively analyzed. The study was a 20 day double blind placebo-controlled, cross-over study of carbamazepine, followed by a twelve week elective double blind second phase, which assessed the reduction of cocaine use among crack users unmotivated for any drug abuse treatment. The motivation for participation in the study was entirely monetary. During the 20 day study, subjects received daily payment in cash to a maximum total of $235 for participation, with a forfeiture of $20 per visit missed. Carbamazepine has indicated some promise in the treatment of cocaine abuse.[30-33]

Each subject admitted to the study met the following rigid criteria: (a) "crack" cocaine use on at least 30 of the previous 100 days; (b) at least 18 years of age; (c) at least eight grade education: (d) no clinically significant medical illness; (e) no seizure disorder; (f) no trauma-induced unconsciousness within the last year; (g) no organic brain syndrome; and, (h) no abnormal laboratory value at screen which could not be explained on the basis of cocaine use.

The 32 subjects who completed the 20 day study were all black males. Their mean age was 33.0 years (SD = 3.9) with a range from 24 to 45 years. Most were unemployed or marginally employed. They lived in transient facilities, rooming houses, shared quarters or on the street. Data for this report was obtained from this group of 32 and from four additional subjects who failed to complete the 20 day study. There is no indication in the literature that carbamazepine or pharmacologically similar drugs cause any myopathy or rhabdomyolysis. Carbamazepine is the most frequently prescribed anticonvulsant in the United States.

These were heavy drug and alcohol users. Thirty three of the 36 subjects reported multiple substance use on more than one day in the 30 days prior to screening visit. Virtually all mixed cocaine use with alcohol or marijuana. Some also used amphetamines, heroin, benzodiazepines, or other substances, along with cocaine. The 36 subjects had reported crack cocaine use on an average of 24 of the 30 days prior to screen, with a mean lifetime cocaine use of 8.1 years (range 9 months to 25 years). They reported alcohol use on an average of 15 of the prior 30 days with a mean lifetime use of 16 years (range 0 to 25 years). Eight subjects had received previous treatment for alcohol abuse; 15 subjects reported previous treatment for drug abuse.

Data was collected at screening, baseline, 20 daily, and 12 subsequent weekly visits. At screening visit, data consisted of: alcohol and drug use history; Addiction Severity Index;[34] medical and psychiatric history; physical examination; blood tests including chemical profile, liver studies, white cell count and differential, thyroid profile, CPK and (if indicated) CKMB; urinalysis and urine drug screen; and electrocardiogram. At all follow up visits, data collected consisted of: vital signs; temperature; repeat chemistry profile (on days 5,10, 15, and 20); WBC with differential (on days 5, 10, 15, and 20); urine analysis for cocaine; signs of obvious trauma; self reported cocaine use (and route); other drug/alcohol use; and adverse effects that might be medication related. Data was obtained during a total of 1126 visits.

RESULTS

A clear elevation in CPK for the overall group was found. Of the 464 CPK results obtained, the mean CPK value was 397 (SD = 784) IU/L with a range of 48 to 13530. Two thirds, 65.5%, of the tests were greater than 200 (upper limit of normal = 198), and 19% were greater than 500 IU/L.

There are many other possible medical explanations for elevated CPK values.[35-38] Therefore, all CPK test results (high or low) which might be otherwise explained, were systematically eliminated. Subjects with medical illness, trauma, and other current abnormal findings had been eliminated by the screening examination. Routine questioning at subsequent visits assessed for any possible episodes of seizures or any adverse symptomatology that might be a result of the drug therapy. During the course of the study, abnormal lab findings identified possible metabolic disorders, such as hypo/hyperthermia (temp); diabetic ketoacidosis (anion gap); hyperosmolar states (glucose/osmolarity); hypokalemia (K^+); hypo/hypernatremia (Na^+); hypophosphatemia (phosphorous). Laboratory-based diagnosis of any intercurrent influenza-like illness without a clinical evaluation required that an algorithm be derived. Any CPK observation was excluded which met two of the following three criteria: WBC $\geq 10 \times 10^9$/L; percent PMN > 75% *or* absolute PMN > 7.5 × 10^9/L; and a temperature > 99 degrees F. This criteria, though adequately sensitive was not specific, and thus would also eliminate CPK tests in which the subject may not have had an influenza-like illness, but might have had some combination of lab findings which could also produce an abnormal CPK.

Using these guidelines, the following CPK results were excluded: one CPK observation was excluded due to a phosphorous value of 1.8 mg/dl; six CPK observations were excluded due to sodium levels below 135 meq/l, (range = 121-134); and 22 observations were excluded on the basis of the influenza algorithm above (maximum WBC = 15.5 × 10 IU/l; maximum temperature = 99.1°, CPK range 137-956 IU/L).

During the 20 day study, there were three reports of reported opiate use and one of amphetamine use; during the 12 week follow up, there were 4 instances of opiate use. Because use of these drugs has been associated with rhabdomyolysis, these CPK results were also deleted from subsequent analyses. Marijuana use, although a frequent occurrence, was not controlled as it has not been described as a cause of RML other than in two case reports when injected.[39] Reanalysis of CPK results with the above 29 observations excluded resulted in a mean of CPK level 400, (s.d. = 791, n = 435), not different from the mean for the entire group.

Alcohol is known to cause an acute and chronic myopathy.[40] The relative contribution of recent alcohol use versus recent cocaine use in raising CPK was therefore assessed by dividing the 435 observations into 4 groups: (a) no alcohol (defined as no reported alcohol use two days prior to daily visit, or no alcohol in the week prior to weekly visit) and no cocaine; (b) alcohol but no cocaine; (c) no alcohol but cocaine; and (d) alcohol and cocaine: For the no alcohol and no cocaine group, the mean CPK was 250 (s.d.= 159, n = 21) with range 101 to 587 IU/L. For the alcohol but no cocaine group, the mean CPK was 290 (s.d. = 190, n = 53) with range 101 to 983

IU/L. For the no alcohol but cocaine group, the mean CPK was 324 (s.d. = 218, n = 63) with range 48 to 870 IU/L. Finally, for the alcohol and cocaine group, the mean CPK was 337 (s.d. = 264, n = 81) with range 48 to 1604. These results are presented in Table 1.

Because the observations are not independent, i.e., the same subjects might have had CPK results in more than one category on different occasions, no statistically valid comparisons across these four groups can be made. By inspection, however, a pattern of increasing muscle toxicity is apparent.

Next, in order to further assess the effect of cocaine alone on CPK, only those CPK results which were drawn on days when urine screens for cocaine were also obtained, were inspected further. There were 215 such observations (alcohol not controlled), with a mean CPK value of 338 (s.d. = 242), and a range of 48-1604. There was no apparent association between the presence of cocaine metabolite in urine and elevated serum CPK values. The mean CPK level with positive cocaine urine was 354 versus mean CPK level with negative cocaine urine, 290. (Chi square could not be used as a test of significance because, again, the observations were not independent). Plotted CPK levels versus quantity of cocaine metabolite demonstrated virtually no relationship (correlation = .014).

Because of the frequently reported use of alcohol during the study by this population, and the known effect of alcohol consumption on CPK, alcohol was then controlled. Alcohol use was excluded based entirely on self reported alcohol/drug use. CPK values for the daily visits when subjects reported alcohol use the day before and/or the day of visit, were excluded. The weekly visit data was analyzed in two ways because weekly alcohol use was reported only as number of days and did not specify recency. First, CPK values were excluded if subjects reported more than 2 days of alcohol use over the prior week (used for analysis #1), and second, if subjects reported any alcohol use over the prior week (analysis #2).

There was no statistically significant relationship (n = 85, correlation = .226, $p > .05$) between CPK and urine cocaine metabolite results in analysis #1. There was, however, a statistically significant relationship found (n = 65, correlation = .318, $p < .05$) between

Table 1

Correlation of Alcohol and Drug Use with CPK Levels

Use	CPK	SD	N	Range
no alc/no coc	250	159	21	101-587
alc/no coc	290	190	53	101-983
no alc/coc	324	218	63	48-870
alc/coc	337	264	81	48-1604

CPK and urine cocaine metabolite results in analysis #2 (no alcohol reported during week prior to each weekly visit).

Thus, "crack" cocaine use in these asymptomatic drug abusers was associated with elevated CPK levels, and, when all other possible causes of elevated CPK levels were controlled, was associated with a positive and significant quantitative effect of cocaine on the CPK level.

DISCUSSION

In our review of the English language literature,[3-5,12-29] a total of 78 anecdotal case reports of RML with cocaine use were found. However, many methodologic problems were also found.

The first problem is the lack of a consistently defined syndrome. Glabow[35] stated that the term "rhabdomyolysis" was preferable to "myoglobinuria"; that clinical symptoms of myalgia and muscle weakness are not discriminatory; that myoglobinuria tests were not clinically practical nor sensitive in RML diagnosis; and that a five-fold (or 500 IU/L) rise in CPK should be considered the sole criteria for RML. Rowland[38] replied that "myoglobinuria" was preferred to "rhabdomyolysis," and that in order to exclude benign elevations in CPK more restrictive criteria should include: myalgias, limb weakness, and, "unequivocally darker than normal urine" for the alert patient; and for the comatose patient, a 100 times normal serum content of sarcoplasmic enzymes.

Many of the 78 cocaine-related literature cases would not meet the second, more restrictive criteria. A major element results from the failure to include all pertinent information in many of the published reports. For example only 44 cases[3,13-15,17-20,22,29] describe clear histories of any myalgias, weakness or flank pain. Nevertheless, the ambiguity of "unequivocally darker than normal," the impracticality of urine myoglobin tests, and the expense of serial enzyme tests for patients with only moderately raised serum levels of sarcoplasmic enzymes suggest that the more rigid criterion will be met more often in specific study paradigms than in clinical work.

In this study, urinalysis was only performed at screen and did not include tests specific for myoglobinuria. Our subjects very rarely reported myalgias or weakness even though they were questioned at each visit regarding any adverse symptomatology. This lack of subject reporting could represent truth, subject non-compliance, or acceptance (by cocaine abusers) of myalgias and weakness as a normal consequence of cocaine abuse. All of these subjects were functioning adults, living independently, with no complaints of illness. For these reasons, this report describes the elevated CPK levels found in these individuals as "asymptomatic."

However, the term "asymptomatic" has further significance than just lack of myalgias and weakness. For the 78 literature cases, cocaine abuse resulted in presentation to a medical facility, often with police escort. Fifty subjects were described as "agitated," "combative," "aggressive," acting in a bizarre manner, or acutely psychotic.[3,4,12,13,15-18,21,23,24] In our study, the subjects reported to the clinic between 9 a.m. and noon, most often before any daily cocaine use. Again, there was no report of adverse symptomatology (such as the above behaviors) nor did observation of the subjects (including those who had used cocaine) indicate abnormal behavior. The 78 reported cases most likely represent either isolated, extreme, cocaine intoxications, or moderate intoxications with serious concomitant medical factors exacerbating the adverse effects of the cocaine.

The problem of adequate controls is an extremely difficult, but a critical issue due to the diverse causes of RML. Authors have previously expressed concerns regarding possible confounding variables in other cases,[14,41] as well as in their own case reports.[5,13-15,17,21] Laboratory identified variables such as chemistry abnormalities are generally easily identified.

However, historical factors are more difficult. As stated, 50 of the 78 literature reports identified aggressive, combative, psychotic behaviors. Another 9 identified episodes of reduced consciousness;[3,15,16,20,25] 8 identified episodes of seizures;[3,12,15] 5 identified hyperthermia;[12,17,18,22] 3 heroin co-abuse;[20,24] and 2 identified alcohol related problems.[18,24]

These variables are difficult to define but should not be overlooked. In this report, there was no history of trauma elicited. Other drug abuse was limited mainly to alcohol. That alcohol is a major factor has been extensively described. One report[42] found a diagnosis of alcoholism in 59% of patients hospitalized for cocaine dependence. In our study, 52 of the 56 screened subjects indicated regular drinking on at least 3 days per week for more than one year duration. Of the 36 subjects followed in our study, 32 met the same use criteria. Their mean self reported alcohol use was 16 years (s.d. = 6, n = 36) with a range of 0 to 25. Thirteen of the 36 subjects had an Addiction Severity Index (ASI) of greater than 5, and 10 had a maximum score of 9. A score greater than 5 indicates a considerable alcohol use problem with treatment indicated.

Finally, a comment on renal failure is warranted. Thirty-six patients of the 78 literature case reports were also given the diagnosis of acute renal failure; seven of these 36 died. During our study, none of the subjects were hospitalized or appeared ill. As a gross predictor of possible oliguria, the CPK values of the subjects who did not produce a urine on the day of a visit were compared with the CPK values for those who did produce a urine sample. For the data from those with no urine samples, the mean CPK was 456 (s.d. = 1061, n = 241) with a range of 54 to 13530 IU/L. For the data from those with urine samples the mean CPK value was 338 (s.d. = 242, n = 215) with range 48 to 1604 IU/L. Furthermore, the mean CPK value for the 47 CPK results over 500 IU/L without urine samples was 1380.5 (s.d. = 2179, range 509 to 13530) almost doubled compared to 724.3 (s.d. = 256, range 508 to 1652) for the 42 CPK results over 500 IU/L with urines.

Several reasons might be postulated for this marked difference. Subjects with higher CPK values (as a result of cocaine use) may have been reticent to disclose their use by producing a urine sample; subjects with high CPK values (as a result of cocaine and/or alcohol use) might have experienced hyperthermia, hypovolemia and/or polyuria resulting in subsequently decreased urine output; or possibly subjects with high CPK values (of any cause) may have experienced brief episodes of oliguria associated with intermittent decreased renal function.

To further evaluate renal function, BUN, creatinine and uric acid values for the group with CPK > 500 IU/L and no urine sample, were analyzed. For these results there were no abnormally high BUN and creatinine values, and only one mildly elevated uric acid value (8.10 mg/dl). Thus, the speculation that the abnormally high CPK values without urine samples possibly represent acute renal damage is not supported by our lab analysis.

Although our data does not indicate renal compromise, the findings may be indirectly significant. The data was collected from September through to November when the potential for developing hyperthermia and/or hypovolemia would be low. This data supports the suggestion that cocaine and alcohol-related rise in serum CPK and myoglobin predisposes an individual to the more serious effects of hyperthermia[23] and/or hypovolemia,[3,17,43] and possibly increases the chance of neuroleptic malignant syndrome if concomitant neuroleptic medications are given. Previously, it has been suggested that neuroleptics may increase or intensify hyperthermia associated with cocaine overdose.[7,44,45] Until disproved, the clinician is urged to promptly evaluate the temperature and volume status of every patient presenting with active cocaine use, and to avoid use of neuroleptic medications.

In summary, it would appear that cocaine use is associated with increased CPK levels in asymptomatic cocaine users. As a clinical observation, it appears that either alcohol or cocaine raises CPK, that cocaine has a greater effect than alcohol, and that both cocaine and alcohol together have a greater effect than either alone. The data further indicates a direct, clinically and statistically significant, relationship between the amount of cocaine metabolite in the urine and the serum CPK level. Although none of the subjects became symptomatic during the study, the precise mechanism causing the 36 cases of acute renal failure (and 13 deaths) in the 78 reviewed literature cases is not clear. Until defined, it is suggested that the clinician make appropriate assessments when evaluating patients that use cocaine. Further investigation is encouraged, but given the lack of precisely detailed case reports and the severity of potential outcome, it is likely that this research will be best accomplished in an animal model.

REFERENCES

1. National Institute on Drug Abuse: Semi-annual Report: Data from the Drug Abuse Warning Network. Series G, Number 19. July-December 1986.

2. Jekel JF, Allen DF, Podlewski H, Clark N, Dean-Patterson S, Cartwright P. Epidemic free-base cocaine abuse: case study from the Bahamas. *Lancet.* 1986, 1:459-62.

3. Roth D, Alarcon FJ, Fernandez JA, Preston RA, Bourgoigne JJ. Acute rhabdomyolysis associated with cocaine intoxication. *N Engl J Med.* 1988,319: 673-7.

4. Jandreski MA, Bermes EW, Leischner R, Kahn SE. Rhabdomyolysis in a case of freebase cocaine ("crack") overdose. *Clin Chem.* 1989, July, 35(7): 1547-9.

5. Merigian KS, Roberts JR. Cocaine intoxication: hyperpyrexia, rhabdomyolysis, and acute renal failure. *Clin Toxicol.* 1987, 25:135-48.

6. Feinman BN. Neurological sequelae of cocaine. *Hosp Pract.* (Off) 1989, Jan 30, 24(14):97-8, 104.

7. Mittleman RE, Wetli CV. Death cause by recreational cocaine use: an update. *JAMA.* 1984, 252:1889-93.

8. Cregler LL, Mark H. Medical complications of cocaine abuse. *N Engl J Med.* 1986, 315:1495-500.

9. Isner JM, Estes NAM III, Thompson PD et al. Acute cardiac events temporally related to cocaine abuse. *N Engl J Med.* 1986, 315:1438-43.

10. Simpson RN, Edwards WD. Pathogenesis of cocaine-induced ischemic heart disease: autopsy findings in a 21 year-old man. *Arch Pathol Lab Med.* 1986, 110:479-84.

11. Lichtenfeld PJ, Rubin DB, Feldman RS. Subarchnoid hemorrhage precipitated by cocaine snorting. *Arch Neurol.* 1984, 41:223-4.

12. Guerin JM, Lustman C, Barbotin-Larricu F. Cocaine-associated acute myoglobinuric renal failure. *South Med J.* 1989, 82(9):1196-7.

13. Parks JM, Reed G, Knochel JP. Cocaine-associated rhabdomyolysis. *Am J Med Sci.* 1989, 297(5):334-6.

14. Rubin RB, Neugarten J. Cocaine-induced rhabdomyolysis masquerading as myocardial ischemia. *Am J Med.* 1989, 86(5):551-3.

15. Singhal P, Horowitz B, Quiñones MC, Sommer M, Faulkner M, Grosser M. Acute renal failure following cocaine abuse. *Nephron.* 1989, 52(1):76-8.

16. Skluth HA, Clark JE, Ehringer GL. Rhabdomyolysis associated with cocaine intoxication. *Drug Intell Clin Pharm.* 1988, 22(10):778-780.

17. Poque VA, Nurse HM. Cocaine-Associated acute myoglobinuric renal failure. *Am J Med.* 1989, 86(2): 183-186.

18. Anand V, Siam G, Stone WJ. Cocaine-associated rhabdomyolysis and acute renal failure. *South Med J.* 1989, 82(1):67-69.

19. Reinhart WH, Stricker H. Rhabdomyolysis after intravenous cocaine. *Am J Med.* 1988, 85(4):579.

20. Herzlich BC, Arsura EL, Pagala M, Grob D. Rhabdomyolysis related to cocaine abuse. *Ann Inter Med.* 1988, 109(4):335-336.

21. Lombard J, Wong B, Young JH. Acute renal failure due to rhabdomyolysis associated with cocaine toxicity. *West J Med.* 1988; 148(4):466-8.

22. Krohn KD, Slowman-Kovacs S, Leapman SB. Cocaine and rhabdomyolysis. *Ann Intern Med.* 1988, 108(4):639-40.

23. Menashe PI, Gottlieb JE. Hyperthermia, rhabdomyolysis, and myoglobinuric renal failure after recreational use of cocaine. *South Med J.* 1988, 81(3):379-81.

24. A case of rhabdomyolysis. *J Tenn Med Assoc.* 1987, 80(10):613.

25. Schwarts JG, McAfee RD. Cocaine and rhabdomyolysis. *J Fam Pract.* 1987, 24(2):209.

26. Flynn JT (ed.). Rhabdomyolysis (clinical conference). *NY State J Med.* 1988, 88(11):582-6.

27. Kassira JP, Kopelman RI. (eds). A defective detective. *Hosp Pract.* Sept. 15, 1986.

28. Barrido DT, Joseph AJ, Rao TKS, Freidman EA Renal disease associated with acute and chronic "crack" abuse. *Kidney Int.* 1988,33:181 Abstract.

29. Zamora-Quezada JC, Dinerman H, Stadecker MJ, Kelly JJ. Muscle and skin infarction after free-basing cocaine (crack). *Ann Intern Med.* 1988, 108(4): 564-566.

30. Halikas JA, Kuhn KL, Carlson GA, Crea F, Crosby RD. The effect of carbamazepine on cocaine use. *The American Journal on Addictions.* Vol. 1(1), Winter 1992, pp. 30-39.

31. Halikas JA, Kemp KD, Kuhn KL, Carlson GA, Crea F. Carbamazepine for cocaine addiction (Letter). *Lancet.* 1989; 8638:623-624.

32. Halikas JA, Kuhn KL. A possible neurophysiological basis of cocaine craving. *Ann Clin Psychiatry* 1990; 2:79-83.

33. Halikas, J.A, Crosby, R.D., Carlson, G.A, Crea, F., Graves, N.M., Bowers, L.D. Cocaine Reduction in Unmotivated Crack Users Using Carbamazepine Versus Placebo in a Short Term Double Blind Crossover Study. *Journal of Clinical Pharmacology and Therapeutics*. Vol. 50(1), pp. 81-95, July, 1991.

34. McLellan AT, Lubersky L, Cacciola J, McGahan P, O'Brien CP. Guide to the Addiction Severity Index: background, administration and field testing results. Washington, DC: National Institute of Drug Abuse. 1988.

35. Gabow, PA, Kaehny, WD, Kelleher SP. The spectrum of rhabdomyolysis. *Medicine*. (Baltimore) 1982, 61:141-152.

36. Milin CJ. Rhabdomyolysis, myoglobinuria and exercise. *Sports Medicine*. 1988, 6:93-106.

37. Knochel JT. Rhabdomyolysis and myoglobinuria. *Ann Rev Med*. 1982, 33:435-443.

38. Rowland LP. Myoglobinuria. *Can J Neurol Sci*. 1984, 11:1-13.

39. Faber SJ, Huertas VE. Intravenously injected marijuana syndrome. *Arch Int Med* 1976, 136:337-339.39.

40. Urbano-Marquez, A, Estruch, R, Navarro-Lopez, F, Grau, JM, Mont, L, Rubin, E. The effects of alcoholism on skeletal and cardiac muscle, *N Engl J Med* 1989; 320:409-415.

41. Howard RC, Kaehny WD. Cocaine and rhabdomyolysis (letter). *Ann Intern Med*. 1989 Jan 1; 110(1):90-1.

42. Weiss RD, Mirin SM, Griffin ML, Michael JL. Psychopathology in Cocaine Abusers. *Journal of Nervous and Mental Disease*. 1988, 176(12):719-725.

43. Bywaters EGL, Stead JK The production of renal failure following injection of solutions containing myohemoglobin. *Q. J. Exp. Physiol*. 1944, 33:53-70.

44. Kosten TR, Kleber HD. Sudden death in cocaine abusers: Relation to neuroleptic malignant syndrome? *Lancet,* 1987, 1:1198-1199.

45. Kosten TR, Kleber HD. Rapid death during cocaine abuse: Variant of neuroleptic malignant syndrome? *American Journal of Alcohol Abuse*. 1988, 12:1-16.

Pathophysiological Effects of Cocaine in Humans: Review of Scientific Issues

David A. Gorelick, MD, PhD

SUMMARY. Almost all data on pathophysiological abnormalities associated with human cocaine use comes from clinical observation and testing of cocaine abusers seeking treatment. Such data are subject to several confounding factors which preclude drawing definitive conclusions about the pathophysiological mechanism for the observed abnormality, its prevalence and prognosis, and individual differences in susceptibility. Confounding factors include the unknown purity of cocaine used, uncertainty as to quantity and duration of cocaine exposure, effects of other substances frequently used by cocaine users, abnormalities associated with drug route of administration and the drug abuse lifestyle, and selection bias. Future studies can address these issues by employing more sophisticated research designs, such as prospective, longitudinal follow-up of large, representative samples of cocaine users, case-control comparisons of well characterized cocaine users with appropriately matched groups, and experimental administration of cocaine under safe, controlled conditions.

Studies of the pathophysiological abnormalities associated with cocaine use follow one of three different research strategies, which vary in their explanatory power. Most published studies to date, including those described in this issue, involve clinical observation and testing of cocaine abusers seeking treatment or volunteering for

David A. Gorelick is Chief, Treatment Branch, Addiction Research Center, National Institute on Drug Abuse, Baltimore, MD and Clinical Professor of Psychiatry, University of Maryland School of Medicine, Baltimore, MD.

Please address correspondence to: Dr. David A. Gorelick, P.O. Box 5180, Baltimore, MD 21224.

research studies. Because of the potentially confounding factors discussed below, data drawn from such naturalistic observation can only suggest, but not definitively prove, a role for cocaine in causing the observed abnormality, nor can such data directly address some important scientific and clinical issues: the pathophysiological mechanism for the abnormality, its prevalence and prognosis (e.g., degree of reversibility), and individual differences in susceptibility (both genetically and environmentally based). The importance of such additional factors (over and above the actions of cocaine, per se) in influencing cocaine-associated abnormalities is illustrated by the poor correlation between cocaine-associated death and blood cocaine concentrations. In one case series of 26 overdose deaths associated only with street cocaine use, blood cocaine levels varied from 0.1-20.9 mg/L.[1]

A second research strategy is case-control studies comparing cocaine users with control subjects matched on relevant variables. By controlling for the matched variables, such studies can help tease out the contribution of confounding factors.[2]

The most definitive results come from studies using experimental administration of cocaine to well characterized subjects, since this allows the greatest control over all relevant factors (including potentially confounding ones). However, this experimental approach tends to be the costliest to carry out and has one theoretical disadvantage. Because of the ethical and practical limitations on exposing human research volunteers to the risk of cocaine, the dose, frequency, and duration of cocaine exposure in experimental studies is unlikely to duplicate the natural exposure of cocaine abusers. Thus, there is always the possibility of a false negative finding, i.e., failure of an experimental study to reproduce a cocaine-associated abnormality found in clinical studies of cocaine abusers.

Use of a variety of research approaches will generate a better understanding of the factors influencing cocaine-associated abnormalities, resulting in a better understanding of the pathophysiological mechanisms involved and improved methods of prevention and treatment. This article will review some of the factors that potentially confound interpretation of clinical data and make suggestions of possible mechanisms for cocaine-related toxicity and avenues for further research.

ESTABLISHING DRUG-EFFECT RELATIONSHIPS

Data from clinical observation and testing usually do not meet unambiguous criteria for establishing a cause-effect relationship between a drug and an observed drug-associated effect. Such criteria would require that (1) the abnormality be absent prior to drug exposure and present after drug exposure; (2) exposure solely to the drug of interest is sufficient to produce the abnormality; and (3) there be a clear dose-effect relationship (in terms of clinical drug abuse data, the greater the exposure to the drug, the greater and/or more frequent the observed abnormality).

The first criterion can be difficult to meet in clinical studies, since subjects are evaluated only after their exposure to cocaine has begun, making it difficult to exclude existence of the abnormality prior to cocaine use. For example, impaired pulmonary function in cocaine users might be due to a pre-existing lung condition such as emphysema or asthma, rather than to cocaine use itself. Careful screening of subjects by history and examination can help reduce this problem.[2] Some factors can provide strong circumstantial evidence against a pre-existing condition as the cause: (1) prompt resolution of the abnormality with abstinence from cocaine; (2) occurrence of a dramatic and otherwise very rare abnormality in the population studied, e.g., stroke or heart attack in young adults.[3]

The second criterion can be equally difficult to meet. Many cocaine-using subjects studied in a variety of settings are using or abusing one or more other substances in addition to cocaine. For example, 86% of cocaine abusers volunteering for a cocaine research project reported current (within last month) use of alcohol, 80% marijuana, 21% opiates, and 13% sedatives.[4] Among cocaine-dependent patients admitted to an inpatient substance abuse treatment program, 85% were also dependent on another substance: 73% on alcohol and 50% on marijuana.[5] In the hospital medical emergency service setting, about one-half of cocaine users report using other drugs (about one-third alcohol).[5,6] Among cocaine-associated deaths reported by medical examiners to the National Institute on Drug Abuse Drug Abuse Warning Network in 1989, only 26.3% involved cocaine alone, while 42.2% involved cocaine plus two or more other drugs.[7] Thus, it would be difficult to draw causal inferences about cocaine-associated medical morbidity and mortality based on these data. Studies of pulmonary function in cocaine abusers are especially confounded by the high prevalence of cigarette and marijuana smoking in such subjects. For example, the heavy cocaine smokers studied by Tashkin et al. (see article in this issue) were 70% current tobacco smokers and 70% current (10%) or former (60%) marijuana smokers.

Even when cocaine is the primary substance used, it is obtained from illicit sources which do not follow any guidelines with regard to purity. Analysis of street cocaine samples reveals a high frequency of both intentional and unintentional adulteration, ranging from naturally occurring cocaine analogues and metabolites (often of unknown biological activity)[8] to inert diluents such as sugars to pharmacologically active substitutions such as other stimulants (e.g., amphetamine, diethylpropion, caffeine, ephedrine, phenylpropanolamine), local anesthetics (e.g., lidocaine), opiates, antipyretics (e.g., quinine, acetaminophen), and CNS depressants (e.g., ketamine, methaqualone).[9]

Any abnormalities observed in illicit cocaine users are potentially the result not only of cocaine, but also of the other substances knowingly used by the subjects, plus the unknown adulterants in the cocaine (and other illicit drugs), plus any interactions among all the substances used. Some of these other substances exert their own pathophysiological effects (some similar to those of cocaine), and thus may contribute to falsely attributing an observed abnormality to cocaine itself. Other substances have pharmacodynamic or pharmacokinetic interactions with cocaine, and thus may produce a type or severity of abnormality that would not occur with cocaine alone. For example, alcohol and marijuana may increase the cardiovascular effects of cocaine in humans,[10,11] and alcohol may potentiate cocaine hepatotoxicity.[12] Sedative drugs which induce the hepatic cytochrome P-450 system may increase the N-demethylation pathway of cocaine metabolism, resulting in increased production of more toxic metabolites such as norcocaine (see below).[13] Concurrent use of alcohol may promote the formation of novel cocaine metabolites,[14,15,16] some of which may be biologically active (e.g., cocaethylene).[14]

Valid dose-response relationships are extremely difficult to derive from clinical data. Subjects' exposure to cocaine, even when studied, is almost exclusively assessed by retrospective self-report, which poses significant problems of reliability and validity.[17,18,19] Even when subjects are motivated to provide accurate data, their memory for past drug use may be impaired, including by the drug use itself. Furthermore, an illicit street drug such as cocaine is rarely sold and used in precisely measured units of defined purity, so that subjects are usually not aware of the precise quantity of drug self-administered. Attempts to objectively confirm cocaine use by assaying body fluids are not very helpful, since the window of detection for cocaine and its metabolites in urine is only several days[20,21] thus at best providing confirmation for only a tiny fraction of the total exposure to cocaine. Should hair analysis for drugs prove valid,[22,23] this would be a useful technique for obtaining objective retrospective longitudinal data on cocaine exposure to correlate with putative cocaine-associated abnormalities. Until valid dose-response relationships are established, it is impossible to answer several clinically relevant questions: Are cocaine-associated abnormalities a continuous function of cocaine exposure? Are there thresholds of exposure for producing cocaine-associated abnormalities? Is there a "safe" level of cocaine use?

OTHER CONFOUNDING FACTORS

Route of cocaine administration and effects of the drug abuse lifestyle are other confounding factors in interpreting clinical studies of cocaine-associated abnormalities. Intravenous cocaine users are subject to the additional adverse medical consequences of needle use, such as contraction of infectious diseases (HIV, hepatitis B) and emboli, while cocaine smokers are subject to the pulmonary effects of inhaled smoke. Cocaine smokers may also be more susceptible to adverse effects for pharmacokinetic reasons. Inhaling cocaine may increase the amount of drug that reaches tissue, since the cocaine is less exposed to enzymatic and nonenzymatic hydrolysis.[20] Direct administration to the lung may potentiate cocaine's effect of inhibiting lung tissue uptake of circulating catecholamines,[24] thus potentiating cocaine's effect on catecholamine activity. All cocaine abusers are likely to suffer from poor nutrition,[25] lack of adequate sleep and exercise, and neglect of personal health. Any or all of these factors could contribute to the abnormalities observed in cocaine users.

Case-control studies comparing cocaine abusers using different routes of administration, or comparing cocaine abusers with non-cocaine using abusers of other drugs can help in distinguishing the pharmacological effects of cocaine itself from the consequences associated with a particular route of administration or a drug abuse lifestyle. This point is illustrated by recent studies of the obstetrical effects of cocaine abuse. Women abusing cocaine during pregnancy not only have higher rates of obstetrical complications than non-drug abusing women, but also higher rates than opiate-dependent women.[26] Since the latter group was also exposed to an illicit drug and drug abuse lifestyle, the significant difference in complications is more confidently attributed to the difference in drug abused, i.e., cocaine vs. opiate.

Studies of clinical samples suffer from substantial selection bias, and so do not provide valid information on the prevalence of cocaine-associated abnormalities, i.e., on the proportion who actually develop the abnormality (numerator) out of the total number of cocaine users (denominator). Both the numerator and the denominator of the prevalence ratio are likely to be falsely estimated. Patients with severer medical abnormalities are more likely to come to medical attention, e.g., the neurological complications of seizure or stroke are more likely to be included in a convenience sample of hospitalized cocaine abusers than are subtler neurological abnormalities. Drug abusers with physical symptoms or associated medical problems may be more likely to seek treatment (and volunteer for related research studies) than those abusers who consider themselves in good physical health.[27,28] Thus, patients with medical abnormalities are likely to be overrepresented in convenience samples of cocaine abusers in treatment. In addition, there may be a publication bias, in that clinical studies reporting abnormalities associated with cocaine use may be more likely to be published than studies reporting no cocaine-associated abnormalities.[29] While the data published to date (including this issue) allow the clinician to counsel cocaine abusers on the range of medical abnormalities associated with cocaine use, they do not allow any precise assessment of risk, i.e., the likelihood that an individual cocaine abuser will suffer a particular medical abnormality.

Another element in assessing risk is the individual's susceptibility to the effects of cocaine. Individual differences in susceptibility probably have genetic, acquired, and environmental components, but this issue has not yet been studied with respect to cocaine. More systematic, large-scale studies with more representative samples (including case-control studies comparing subjects with and without cocaine-associated abnormalities) are needed to address this issue.

One possible susceptibility factor is the metabolism of cocaine. In humans, the major (90-95%) metabolic pathway is hydrolysis to inactive metabolites, both nonenzymatically (at physiological pH) and enzymatically catalyzed by butyrylcholinesterase (also known as pseudo-, serum, or plasma cholinesterase) found in plasma, liver, pancreas, and other tissues.[20,30] A minor pathway, more prominent in rodents, is N-demethylation to norcocaine by the hepatic cytochrome P-450 system.[20] As might be expected, the degree of cocaine N-demethylation is inversely correlated with plasma cholinesterase activity.[31] Since norcocaine is biologically active as a local anesthetic and its metabolites are hepatotoxic[20,32] level of cholinesterase activity could influence cocaine hepatotoxicity. This relationship is supported by the fact that cholinesterase inhibitors enhance cocaine hepatotoxicity in animals.[32]

Human plasma cholinesterase activity is under genetic control, with four alleles identified for the primary gene.[30,33] Up to 4% of the population has abnormal variants of the enzyme, the vast majority exhibiting about 50% of normal activity, although one very rare genotype exhibits two- to three-fold increased activity.[30,33] There is also substantial physiological variation in cholinesterase activity, with infants, women (especially pregnant women), the elderly, and liver disease patients tending to have lower activity.[30] Individuals with lower enzyme activity could be more susceptible to cocaine effects, and at greater risk for hepatotoxicity (from increased norcocaine production), and perhaps other toxicities, from cocaine use.

No clinical studies have yet addressed the relationship between plasma cholinesterase activity and response to cocaine.

The reversibility of cocaine-associated abnormalities is another important issue which has not yet been adequately studied. This is clinically relevant in terms of counseling patients on their prognosis with continued abstinence from cocaine use. Some clinical data already suggest that physiological abnormalities associated with cocaine use can resolve with abstinence. For example, the myocardial ischemia detected on ambulatory Holter monitoring of cocaine abusers entering treatment seems to disappear over several weeks of abstinence in most patients.[34] With respect to pulmonary function, the study by Tashkin et al.[2] is collecting follow-up data to address the issue of reversibility. One small study has already found that both self-reported pulmonary symptoms and abnormal lung sounds decrease over 5 days of abstinence.[35] However, not all abnormalities decreased to the same extent, highlighting the possibility of differential recovery from cocaine-associated abnormalities.

MECHANISMS OF ACTION

The known pharmacological actions of cocaine can plausibly account for the pathophysiological abnormalities found in cocaine abusers. Cocaine acts as a local anesthetic, presumably by blocking sodium channels in the nerve membrane.[21] It also stimulates central and peripheral catecholaminergic (sympathetic) activity. This increased catecholaminergic activity may occur from several mutually reinforcing mechanisms:[21,24] (1) blockade of presynaptic catecholamine (especially dopamine) reuptake, leaving more neurotransmitter in the synapse; (2) release of catecholamines, especially from the adrenal medulla; (3) decreased clearance of circulating catecholamines in the lung; (4) sensitization of catecholamine receptors; and (5) cocaine-induced steroid hormone release, resulting in steroid potentiation of catecholamine action. The physiological consequences of these cocaine actions presumably result in the medical abnormalities found in cocaine abusers.

Cocaine, like other local anesthetics, produces kindling in animals, i.e., a sensitization of certain areas of the brain (especially the limbic system) so that repeated low intensity electrical or chemical stimulation, which previously was below the threshold for evoking a response, now evokes a strong response, e.g., a seizure. Cocaine-induced kindling, although never directly demonstrated in humans, could explain some cocaine-associated abnormalities, e.g., tinnitus, seizures, sudden death,[36] especially those occurring in intermittent or infrequent cocaine users. Kindling has also been hypothesized as the mediator of some psychological manifestations of cocaine use, such as the panic attacks reported in cocaine users and cocaine craving.[36,37]

Explanations for some of the puzzling observations relating kindling and the psychoactive properties of cocaine and other local anesthetics would greatly improve our understanding of the pathophysiology of cocaine effects. For example, at equally local anesthetic doses, cocaine-stimulated seizures are much more lethal than lidocaine-stimulated seizures.[36] While lidocaine is as potent a local anesthetic as cocaine, and both are more potent than procaine, it is procaine and cocaine which have similar psychoactive properties (e.g., both self-administered by animals, often cannot be distinguished from one another in animal and human drug discrimination studies), while lidocaine does not.[21,36]

The vascular consequences of cocaine's actions could account for many of the cardiovascular, pulmonary, and neurological abnormalities found in cocaine abusers. Sympathetic (alpha-1 adrenergic) stimulation would lead to vasoconstriction and vasospasm.[38] Cocaine itself may also exacerbate the effects of vasoconstriction and vasospasm by enhancing hemostasis by several mechanisms, including increased platelet aggregability, increased thromboxane production, and decreased endothelial prostacycline release.[34] In the systemic circulation, these cocaine effects would raise blood pressure, increasing strain on the heart. In the coronary circulation, they could cause myocardial ischemia,[36,39,40] potentially resulting in infarction.[38] In the lungs, they could decrease pulmonary blood flow,[41] resulting in decreased gas diffusion capacity. In the cerebral circulation, they could cause cerebral ischemia or hemorrhage, resulting in seizures or stroke.[3] In the hepatic circulation, the decreased blood flow could lead to reduced clearance of endogenous compounds and drugs.[13]

Direct tissue effects of cocaine may also cause some abnormalities. For example, seven cases of cocaine users presenting with frank congestive heart failure have been reported, with no evidence of another etiology and cardiac biopsy showing only minimal myocarditis or interstitial fibrosis.[42] A direct myocardial depressant effect of cocaine, as recently demonstrated experimentally in dogs[43] could explain these cases. Similarly, direct damage by cocaine (especially smoked cocaine) to pulmonary gas exchange surfaces could explain reports of impaired gas diffusing capacity in cocaine abusers.[44] However, in both organs, direct toxicity from contaminants in the cocaine used can not be ruled out. Variations in the purity (and route of administration) of the illicit cocaine used by subjects at different time periods in different geographic areas could account for varying results in different studies.

TREATMENT IMPLICATIONS

A better understanding of the pathophysiological mechanisms of cocaine-associated medical abnormalities should lead to improved treatment for these consequences of cocaine abuse. Initial work in animals with adrenergic antagonists (both alpha and beta) and with calcium channel blockers suggests that such medications may be useful in ameliorating or blocking some pathophysiological effects of cocaine on the nervous system,[45,46] cardiopulmonary system[45,47,48] and the liver.[49]

The hypothesis that kindling mediates psychological effects of cocaine has led to the use of the anti-convulsant carbamazepine (Tegretol), which retards development of cocaine-kindled seizures in rodents,[50] as a treatment for cocaine abuse. While initial open label clinical experience has been successful,[37,51] controlled, double-blind studies remain to be done. One intriguing pharmacological question about the carbamazepine-cocaine interaction is why carbamazepine influences cocaine-kindled seizures only when administered chronically in the diet, but not when administered parenterally, even on a daily basis.[52]

CONCLUSIONS

In summary, the clinical studies reported in this issue and elsewhere suggest the wide range of medical consequences associated with cocaine, but leave many important clinical and scientific issues unresolved. Further research is needed to establish a direct cause-effect relationship between cocaine use and the observed abnormalities in patients and to determine the mechanism of action, to identify particular patterns of cocaine use and other characteristics (both genetic and environmental) that influence vulnerability to abnormalities, and to develop improved treatments to ameliorate the pathophysiological effects of cocaine use.

Future studies will need to employ more sophisticated research designs in order to satisfactorily address these issues. Such studies should include (1) prospective, longitudinal follow-up of large samples of cocaine users more representative of age, ethnicity, gender, and variations in use patterns, including community-living subjects not in medical or drug abuse treatment; (2) case-control studies comparing well characterized cocaine users with a variety of appropriate comparison groups, e.g., intravenous vs. smoked cocaine users, cocaine abusers vs. non-cocaine drug abusers; and (3) experimental studies in which subjects' cocaine exposure is known precisely because the cocaine is administered under experimenter control. The latter type of study, although subject to ethical and practical limitations of design, will be crucial in exploring the mechanisms by which cocaine produces pathophysiological abnormalities and in developing treatments for these.

REFERENCES

1. Mittleman RE, Wetli, CV, Death caused by recreational cocaine use: an update. *JAMA* 1984; 252:1989-1893.

2. Tashkin DP, Gorelick, DA, Khalsa, H. and Simmons et al. Respiratory effects of cocaine freebasing among habitual cocaine users. *J Addictive Diseases* (1992) 11(4):61-72.

3. Miller BL, Mena, Giombetti, Villanueva-Meyer et al. Neuropsychiatric effects of cocaine: SPECT measurements. *J Addictive Diseases* (1992) 11(4):49-60.

4. Schuster CR, and Fischman, NW, Characteristics of humans volunteering for a cocaine research project. *NIDA Res. Monogr.* 1985; 61: 158-170.

5. Miller NS, Golds, MS, and Belkin, BM, The diagnosis of alcohol and cannabis dependence in cocaine dependence. *Adv. Alcohol & Substance Abuse* 1990; 8:33-42.

6. Brody SL, Slovis, CM, Wrenn, KD, Cocaine-related medical problems: consecutive series of 233 patients. *Amer. J. Med.* 1990; 88:325-331.

7. National Institute on Drug Abuse. *Data from the Drug Abuse Warning Network (DAWN): Annual Data 1989.* 1990; Statistical Series, Series 1, No. 9.

8. Noggle FT, and Clark, CR, Liquid chromatographic identification of *cis*- and *trans*- cinnamoylcocaine in illicit cocaine. *J. Assoc. Off. Anal. Chem.* 1982; 65:756-761.

9. Renfroe CL, and Messinger, TA. Street drug analysis: an eleven year perspective on illicit drug alteration. *Seminars Adol. Med.* 1985; 1:247-257.

10. Lynn M, Higgins, ST Bickel, WK, Hughes, JR. et al. Behavioral and cardiovascular effects of cocaine and alcohol combinations in humans. Presented at Committee on Problems of Drug Dependence annual meeting, Richmond, VA, June 1990.

11. Foltin RW, Fischman, MW, Pedroso, JJ, and Pearlson, GD. Marijuana and cocaine interactions in humans: cardiovascular consequences. *Pharmacol Biochem Behav* 1987; 28:459-464.

12. Conners S, Rankin, DR, Krumdieck, CL, and Brendel, K. Interactive toxicity of cocaine with phenobarbital, morphine and ethanol in organ cultured human and rat liver slices. *Proc. West. Pharmacol. Soc.* 1989; 32:205-208.

13. Shuster L, Garhar, CA, Powers, J, Grunfeld, Y, and Kanel, G. Hepatotoxicity of Cocaine. *NIDA Res. Monogr.* 1988; 88:250-275.

14. Hearn WL, Flynn, DD, Hime, GWR, Stefan et al. Cocaethylene: a unique cocaine metabolite displays high affinity for the dopamine transporter. *J. Neurochem* 1991; Vol. 56, in press.

15. Rafla FK, and Epstein, RL. Identification of cocaine and its metabolites in human urine in the presence of ethyl alcohol. *J. Anal. Toxicol.* 1979; 3:59-63.

16. Smith RM, Ethyl esters of arylhydroxy- and arylhydroxymeth- oxycocaines in the urines of simultaneous cocaine and ethanol users. *J. Anal. Toxicol.* 1984; 8:38-42.

17. Aiken LS, Retrospective self-reports by clients differ from original reports: implications for the evaluation of drug treatment programs. *Int. J. Addict.* 1986; 21:767-788.

18. Magura S, and Lipton, DS. The accuracy of drug use monitoring in methadone treatment. *J. Drug Issues* 1988; 18:317-326.

19. Stephens R, The truthfulness of addict respondents in research projects. *Int. J. Addict.* 1972; 7:549-558.

20. Inaba T, Cocaine: pharmacokinetics and biotransformation in man. *Can. J. Physiol.* 1989; 67:1154-1157.

21. Johanson CE, and Fischman, MW, The pharmacology of cocaine related to its abuse. *Pharmacol. Rev.* 1989; 41:3-52.

22. Bailey DN, Drug screening in an unconventional matrix; hair analysis. *JAMA* 1989; 262:3331.

23. Graham K, Koren, G, Klein, J, Schneiderman, J et al. Determination of gestational cocaine exposure by hair analysis. *JAMA* 1989; 262:3328-3330.

24. Wilkins JN, Brain, lung and heart interactions with cocaine and cocaine-induced catecholamines. *J Addictive Diseases* (1992) 11(4): 9-19.

25. Mohs ME, Watson, RR, and Leonard, GT, Nutritional effects of marijuana, heroin, cocaine, and nicotine. *J. Am Diet Assoc.* 1990; 90:1261-1267.

26. Ryan L, Ehrlich, S, and Finnegan, L, Cocaine abuse in pregnancy: effects on the fetus and newborn. *Neurotoxicol Teratol.* 1987; 9:295-299.

27. Chitwood DD, and Morningstar, PC, Factors which differentiate cocaine users in treatment from nontreatment users. *Int. J Addict.* 1985; 20:449-459.

28. Rounsaville BJ, and Kleber, HD. Untreated opiate addicts. *Arch. Gen. Psychiatry* 1985; 42:1072-1077.

29. Koren G, Shear, H, Graham, K, and Einarson, T. Bias against the null hypothesis; the reproductive hazards of cocaine. *Lancet* 1989; II: 1440-1442.

30. Trundle D, and Marcial, G. Detection of Cholinesterase Inhibition. The Significance of Cholinesterase Measurements. *Ann. Clin. Lab. Sci.* 1988; 18:345-351.

31. Inaba T, Stewart DJ, and Kalow, W. Metabolism of cocaine in man. *Clin. Pharmacol. Ther.* 1978; 23:547-552.

32. Freeman RW, and Harbison, RD. The role of benzoylmethylecgonine in cocaine-induced hepatotoxicity. *J. Pharmacol. Exp. Ther.* 1981; 218:558-567.

33. La Du BN, Genetic factors modifying drug metabolism and drug response. In La Du, BN, Mandel, HG, and Way, EL, (eds.). *Fundamentals of Drug Metabolism and Drug Disposition.* Baltimore, MD: Williams & Wilkins, 1971; pp 308-327.

34. Nademanee K, Gorelick, DA, Josephson, MA, Ryan, MA, Wilkins, JN et al. Myocardial ischemia during cocaine withdrawal. *Ann. Intern. Med,* 1989; 111: 876-880.

35. Delbono EA, O'Brien, K. and Murphy, Raymond LN. Lung sound abnormalities in cocaine freebasers. *Substance Abuse* 1989; 10:201-208.

36. Post RM, and Weiss, SRM. Psychomotor stimulant vs. local anesthetic effects of cocaine: Role of behavioral sensitization and kindling. *NIDA Res. Monogr.* 1988; 88:217-238.

37. Halikas J, Kuhn, KL, and Maddux, TL. Reduction of cocaine use among methadone maintenance patients using concurrent carbamazepine maintenance. *Ann. Clin. Psychi.* 1990; 2:3-6, and 2:79-83.

38. Nademanee K, Cardiovascular effects and toxicities of Cocaine. *J. Addictive Diseases* (1992) 11(4):73-84.

39. Lange RA, Cigarroa, RG, Yancy, CW, Willard, JE, et al. Cocaine-induced coronary-artery vasoconstriction. *New England J. Med.* 1989; 321:1558-1562.

40. Vitullo JC, Karam, R, Mekhail, N, Wicker, P et al. Cocaine-induced small vessel spasm in isolated rat hearts. *Am. J. Pathol.* 1989; 135:85-91.

41. Murray R, Smialek, J, Golle, M. and Albin R. Pulmonary vascular abnormalities in cocaine users. *Amer. Rev. Respiratory Dis.* 1988; 137(4 Suppl.) :459.

42. Peng SK, French, WJ, and Pelikan, PCD. Direct cocaine cardiotoxicity demonstrated by endomyocardial biopsy. *Arch Pathol Lab Med* 1989; 113:842-845.

43. Abel FL, Wilson, SP, Zhao, RR and Fennell, WH. Cocaine depresses the canine myocardium. *Circulatory Shock* 1989; 28:309-319.

44. Weiss, RD, Tilles, DS, Goldenheim, PD, and Mirin, SM. Decreased single breath carbon monoxide diffusing capacity in cocaine freebase smokers. *Drug Alcohol Dependence* 1987; 19:271-276.

45. Rossetti ZL, Pani, L, Kuzmin, A, Carboni, S, and Gessa, GL. Dihydropyridine calcium antagonists prevent cocaine, but not amphetamine, induced dopamine release and motor activity in rats. *Acta. Physiol. Hung.* 1990; 75 (Suppl.) 249-250.

46. Trouve R, Nahas, GG, Manager, WM, Vinyard, C, and Goldberg, S. Interactions of nimodipine and cocaine on endogenous catecholamines in the squirrel monkey. *Proc. Soc. Exp. Bio. Med.* 1990; 193:171-175.

47. Robin ED, Wong, RJ. and Ptashne, KA. Increased lung water and ascites after massive cocaine overdosage in mice and improved survival related to beta-adrenergic blockage. *Ann. Intern. Med.* 1989; 110:202-207.

48. Tella, SR, Schindler, CW, and Goldberg, SR. The role of central and autonomic neural mechanisms in the cardiovascular effects of cocaine in conscious squirrel monkeys. *J. Pharmacol. Exp. Ther.* 1990; 252:491-499.

49. James RC, Schiefer, MA, Roberts, SM, and Harbison, RD. Antagonism of cocaine-induced hepatotoxicity by the alpha adrenergic antagonists phentolamine and yohimbine. *J. Pharmacol. Exp. Ther.* 1987; 242:726-732.

50. Weiss, SRB, Post, RM, Costello, M, Nutt, DJ et al. Carbamazepine retards the development of cocaine-kindled seizures but not sensitization to cocaine-induced hyperactivity. *Neuropsychopharmacol.* 1990; 3:273-281.

51. Halikas J, Kemp, K, Kuhn, K et al. Carbamazepine for cocaine addiction? *Lancet* 1989; 1:623-624.

52. Weiss, SRB, Post, RM, Szele, F, Woodward, R et al. Chronic carbamazepine inhibits the development of local anesthetic seizures kindled by cocaine and lidocaine. *Brain Res.* 1989; 497:72-79.

SELECTIVE GUIDE TO CURRENT REFERENCE SOURCES ON TOPICS DISCUSSED IN THIS ISSUE

Cocaine: Physiological and Physiopathological Effects

Lynn Kasner Morgan, MLS
James E. Raper, Jr., MSLS

Each issue of *Journal of Addictive Diseases* features a section offering suggestions on where to look for further information on included topics. In this issue, our intent is to guide readers to selective substantive sources of current information on the physiological and physiopathological effects of cocaine.

Some published reference works utilize designated terminology (controlled vocabularies) which must be used to find material on topics of interest. For these, a sample of available search terms has

Lynn Kasner Morgan is Assistant Professor of Medical Education, Assistant Dean for Information Resources and Systems, and Director of the Gustave L. and Janet W. Levy Library of the Mount Sinai Medical Center, Inc. James Raper is an instructor in Medical Education and Assistant Director for Technical Services at Mount Sinai, One Gustave L. Levy Place, New York, NY 10029-6574.

been indicated to assist the reader in accessing suitable sources for his/her purposes. Other reference tools use keywords or free-text terms from the title of the document, the abstract, and the name of any responsible agency or conference. In searching using keywords, be sure to look under all possible synonyms to retrieve the concept in question.

An asterisk (*) appearing before a published source indicates that all or part of that source is in machine-readable form and can be accessed through an online database search. Database searching is recommended for retrieving sources of information that coordinate multiple variables, concepts or subject areas. Most health sciences libraries offer database services which can include mediated online searching, access to locally mounted datafiles, front-end software packages, and CD-ROM technology. Searching can also be done from one's office or home with subscriptions to database services and microcomputers equipped with modems.

Readers are encouraged to consult their librarians for further assistance before undertaking research on a topic.

Suggestions regarding the content and organization of this section are welcome and should be sent to the authors.

1. INDEXING AND ABSTRACTING SOURCES

Place of publication, publisher, start date, frequency of publication, and brief descriptions are noted.

**Biological Abstracts* (1926-) and *Biological Abstracts/RRM* (v.18, 1980-). Philadelphia, BioSciences Information Service, semimonthly. Reports on worldwide research in the life sciences.

See: Concept headings for abstracts, such as behavioral biology, pharmacology, psychiatry, public health, and toxicology sections.

See: Keyword-in-context subject index.

**Chemical Abstracts*. Columbus, Ohio, American Chemical Society, 1907- , weekly. A key to the world's literature of chemistry and chemical engineering, including journal articles, patents, reviews, technical reports, monographs, conference proceedings, symposia, dissertations, and books.

See: *Index Guide* for cross-referencing and indexing policies.

See: *General Subject Index* terms, such as cardiovascular agents, drug dependence, drug-drug interactions, drug tolerance, respiratory center, respiratory distress syndrome, respiratory tract, sleep.

See: Keyword subject indexes.

**Criminal Justice Periodical Index*. Ann Arbor, Mich., Indexing Services, University Microfilms, 1975-, 3 times per year, including annual cumulation. Covers more than 100 English-language journals in criminology, including drug abuse.

See: Keyword subject index.

**Dissertation Abstracts International. Section B. The Sciences and Engineering*. Ann Arbor, Mich., University Microfilms, v. 30, 1969/70- , monthly. Includes author-prepared abstracts of doctoral dissertations from 500 participating institutions throughout North America and the world. A separate section contains European dissertations.

See: Keyword subject index.

**Excerpta Medica*. Amsterdam, The Netherlands, Excerpta Medica Foundation, 1947- , 45 subject sections. A major abstracting service covering more than 4,300 biomedical journals. The abstracts, including English summaries for non-English-language articles, appear in one or more of the published subject sections, excluding Section 37, *Drug Literature Index*, and Section 38, *Adverse Reactions Titles*, which are indexes only. Each of the sections has a comprehensive subject index. Since 1978 all the *Excerpta Medica* sections have been available for computer searching in the integrated online file, EMBASE.

Particularly relevant to the topics in this issue are Section 40, *Drug Dependence, Alcohol Abuse and Alcoholism*; and the sections that have addiction, alcoholism, or drug subdivisions: Section 130, *Clinical Pharmacology*; Section 30, *Pharmacology*; Section 32, *Psychiatry*; and Section 17, *Public Health, Social Medicine and Epidemiology*.

**Index Medicus* (includes *Bibliography of Medical Reviews*). Bethesda, Md., National Library of Medicine, 1960- , monthly, with annual cumulations. Published as author and subject indexes to more than 3,800 journals in the biomedical sciences. Subject headings are based on the controlled vocabulary or thesaurus, *Medical Subject Headings* (MeSH). Since 1966 it has been produced from the MEDLARS database, which provides more comprehensive retrieval, including keyword access and English-language abstracts, than its printed counterparts: *Index Medicus*, *International Nursing Index*, and *Index to Dental Literature*. As an example of enhanced online retrieval, the subheading "physiopathology" can be coordinated with the major heading "substance abuse" to search drug-induced abnormal organ functions.

See: *MeSH* terms, such as affect; brain diseases; cardiovascular diseases; cerebrovascular disorders; catecholamines; cocaine; creatine kinase; drug hypersensitivity; drug interactions; drug resistance; drug therapy; electroencephalography; emotions; heart diseases; lung diseases; mental disorders; narcotics; pharmacology; rehabilitation; respiration disorders; sleep; sleep stages; sleep disorders; substance abuse; substance withdrawal syndrome; substance dependence; substance use disorders; tomography, emission-computed, single-photon; toxicology.

Index to Scientific Reviews. Philadelphia, Institute for Scientific Information, 1974- , semiannual.

See: Permuterm keyword subject index.

See: Citation index.

**International Pharmaceutical Abstracts*. Washington, D.C., American Society of Hospital Pharmacists, 1964- , semimonthly. A key to the world's literature of pharmacy.

See: IPA subject terms, such as cocaine, controlled substance analogs, dependence, drug abuse.

**Psychological Abstracts.* Washington, D.C., American Psychological Association, 1927- , monthly. A compilation of nonevaluative summaries of the world's literature in psychology and related disciplines.

See: Index terms, such as addiction, central nervous system, cocaine, drug abuse, drug addiction, drug dependency, drug interactions, drug usage, respiration, sleep.

**Public Affairs Information Service Bulletin.* New York, Public Affairs Information Service, v. 55, 1969- , semimonthly. An index to informational resources in the field of public affairs and public policy published throughout the world.

See: *PAIS* subject headings, such as cocaine, drug abuse, drug addicts, drugs, narcotics.

**Science Citation Index.* Philadelphia, Institute for Scientific Information, 1961- , bimonthly.

See: Permuterm keyword subject index.

See: Citation index.

**Social Planning/Policy & Development Abstracts.* San Diego, Calif., Sociological Abstracts, Inc., v. 6, 1984- , semiannual.

See: Thesaurus and descriptors listed under *Sociological Abstracts.*

**Social Work Research and Abstracts.* New York, National Association of Social Workers, v. 13, 1977- , quarterly.

See: Fields of service sections, such as health and health care, substance use and abuse/alcoholism.

See: Subject index.

**Sociological Abstracts.* San Diego, Calif., Sociological Abstracts, Inc., 1952- , 6 times per year. A collection of nonevaluative abstracts which reflect the world's serial literature in sociology and related disciplines.

See: *Thesaurus of Sociological Indexing Terms.*

See: Descriptors such as cocaine, drug abuse, drug addiction, drug use, substance abuse.

Substance Abuse Index and Abstracts: A Guide to Drug, Alcohol and Tobacco Research. New York, Scientific DataLink, 1989- , annual with supplements. A multidisciplinary guide to the literature on psychoactive substance use and abuse, prevention, treatment and control.

See: Subject index.

2. CURRENT AWARENESS PUBLICATIONS

*Current Contents: Clinical Medicine. Philadelphia, Institute for Scientific Information, v. 15, 1987- , weekly.

See: Keyword index.

**Current Contents: Life Sciences.* Philadelphia, Institute for Scientific Information, v. 10, 1967- , weekly.

See: Keyword index.

**Current Contents: Social & Behavioral Sciences.* Philadelphia, Institute for Scientific Information, v. 6, 1974- , weekly.

See: Keyword index.

3. BOOKS

Andrews, Theodora. *A Bibliography of Drug Abuse, Including Alcohol and Tobacco.* Littleton, Colo., Libraries Unlimited, 1977- .

Andrews, Theodora. *Guide to the Literature of Pharmacy and the Pharmaceutical Sciences.* Littleton, Colo., Libraries Unlimited, 1986.

Cocaine: An Annotated Bibliography. Jackson, Research Institute of Pharmaceutical Sciences, University of Mississippi and University Press of Mississippi, c1988.

**Medical and Health Care Books and Serials in Print: An Index to Literature in the Health Sciences.* New York, R.R. Bowker Co., annual.

See: Library of Congress subject headings, such as cocaine, drug abuse, drugs, narcotic habit, rehabilitation.

**National Library of Medicine Current Catalog.* Bethesda, Md., National Library of Medicine, 1966- , quarterly, with annual cumulations.

See: *MeSH* terms as noted in Section 1 under *Index Medicus.*

Page, Penny B. *Alcohol Use and Alcoholism: A Guide to the Literature.* New York, Garland Publishing, 1986.

World Health Organization Catalogue: New Books. Geneva, World Health Organization, semiannual (supplements *World Health Organization Publications* and includes periodicals).

4. U.S. GOVERNMENT PUBLICATIONS

**Monthly Catalog of United States Government Publications.* Washington, D.C., U.S. Government Printing Office, 1895- , monthly.

See: Following agencies: Alcohol, Drug Abuse and Mental Health Administration; Centers for Disease Control; Food and Drug Administration; National Center for Health Statistics; National Institute of Mental Health; National Institute on Drug Abuse; National Institutes of Health.

See: Subject headings, derived chiefly from the Library of Congress, such as cocaine, drug abuse, drug habit, drug interactions, drug utilization, drug dependence, drugs, narcotics, pharmacology.

See: Title index.

5. ONLINE BIBLIOGRAPHIC DATABASES

Only those databases which have no print counterparts are included in this section. Print sources which have online database equivalents are noted throughout this guide by the asterisk (*) which appears before the title. If you do not have direct access to these databases, consult your librarian for assistance.

ASI: AMERICAN STATISTICS INDEX (Congressional Information Services, Inc., Washington, D.C.).

Use: Keywords.

DRUG INFORMATION FULLTEXT (American Society of Hospital Pharmacists, Bethesda, Md.).

Use: Keywords.

DRUGINFO AND ALCOHOL USE AND ABUSE (Hazelden Foundation, Center City, Minn., and Drug Information Service Center, College of Pharmacy, University of Minnesota, Minneapolis, Minn.).

Use: Keywords.

FAMILY RESOURCES DATABASE (National Council on Family Relations and Inventory of Marriage and Family Literature Project, Minneapolis, Minn.).

Use: Keywords.

LEXIS (Mead Data Central, Inc., Dayton, Ohio).

Use: Keywords.

MAGAZINE INDEX (Information Access Co., Belmont, Calif.).

Use: Keywords.

MEDICAL AND PSYCHOLOGICAL PREVIEWS: MPPS (BRS Bibliographic Retrieval Services, Inc., McLean, Va.).

Use: Keywords.

MENTAL HEALTH ABSTRACTS (IFI/Plenum Data Co., Alexandria, Va.).

Use: Keywords.

NATIONAL NEWSPAPER INDEX (Information Access Co., Belmont, Calif.).

Use: Keywords.

NTIS (National Technical Information Service, U.S. Dept. of Commerce, Springfield, Va.).

Use: Keywords.

PSYCINFO (American Psychological Association, Washington, D.C.).

Use: Keywords.

WESTLAW (West Publishing Co., St. Paul, Minn.).

Use: Keywords.

6. HANDBOOKS, DIRECTORIES, GRANT SOURCES, ETC.

Annual Register of Grant Support. Wilmette, Ill., National Register Pub. Co., annual.

See: Internal medicine, medicine; pharmacology; psychiatry, psychology, mental health sections.

See: Subject index.

**Biomedical Index to PHS-Supported Research*. Bethesda, Md., National Institutes of Health, Division of Research Grants, annual.

See: Subject index.

**Database Directory*. White Plains, N.Y., Knowledge Industry Publications in cooperation with the American Society for Information Science, annual.

See: Subject index.

**Directory of Online Databases* (includes *Online Databases in the Medical and Life Sciences*). New York, Cuadra/Elsevier, quarterly.

See: Subject index.

Directory of Research Grants. Phoenix, Ariz., Oryx Press, annual.

See: Subject index terms, such as drug abuse.

**Encyclopedia of Associations*. Detroit, Gale Research Co., annual (occasional supplements between editions).

See: Subject index.

Encyclopedia of Information Systems and Services. Detroit, Gale Research Co., annual (updated by New Information Systems and Services).

Evans, Glen [and others]. *The Encyclopedia of Drug Abuse*. 2nd ed., rev. and expanded. New York, Facts on File Pub., c1991.

**Foundation Directory*. New York, The Foundation Center, biennial (updated between editions by *Foundation Directory Supplement*).

See: Index of foundations.

See: Index of foundations by state and city.

See: Index of donors, trustees, and administrators.

See: Index of fields of interest.

**Health Hotlines: Toll-Free Numbers from DIRLINE*. Bethesda, Md., National Library of Medicine, 1990.

Roper, Fred W. and Jo Anne Boorkman. *Introduction to Reference Sources in the Health Sciences*. 2nd ed. Chicago, Medical Library Association, c1984.

The SALIS Directory: Substance Abuse Librarians and Information Specialists 2nd ed. Berkeley, Calif., Alcohol Research Group, Medical Research Institute of San Francisco and University of California, Berkeley, 1991.

Statistics Sources. Detroit, Gale Research Co., annual.

7. JOURNAL LISTINGS

**Ulrich's International Periodicals Directory, Now Including Irregular Serials & Annuals.* New York, R. R. Bowker Co., annual (updated between editions by *Ulrich's Update*).

See: Subject categories, such as drug abuse and alcoholism, medical sciences, pharmacy and pharmacology, psychology.

8. AUDIOVISUAL PROGRAMS

The Directory of Medical Video Programs. Hawthorne, N.J., Ridge Publishing Co., 1990.

**National Library of Medicine Audiovisuals Catalog.* Bethesda, Md., National Library of Medicine, 1977- , quarterly, with annual cumulations.

See: *MeSH* terms as noted in Section 1 under *Index Medicus.*

Patient Education Sourcebook. 2 v. Saint Louis, Mo., Health Sciences Communications Association, c1985-90.

See: *MeSH* terms as noted in Section 1 under *Index Medicus.*

9. GUIDES TO UPCOMING MEETINGS

Scientific Meetings. San Diego, Calif., Scientific Meetings Publications, quarterly.

See: Subject indexes.

See: Association listing.

World Meetings: Medicine. New York, Macmillan Pub. Co., quarterly.

See: Keyword index.

See: Sponsor directory and index.

World Meetings: Outside United States and Canada. New York, Macmillan Pub. Co., quarterly.

See: Keyword index.

See: Sponsor directory and index.

World Meetings: United States and Canada, New York, Macmillan Pub. Co., quarterly.

See: Keyword index.

See: Sponsor directory and index.

10. PROCEEDINGS OF MEETINGS

**Conference Papers Index.* Louisville, Ky., Data Courier, v.6, 1978- , monthly.

**Directory of Published Proceedings. Series SEMT. Science/Engineering/Medicine/Technology.* White Plains, N.Y., InterDok Corp., v. 3, 1967- , monthly, except July-August, with annual cumulations.

**Index to Scientific and Technical Proceedings.* Philadelphia, Institute for Scientific Information, 1978- , monthly with semiannual cumulations.

11. SPECIALIZED RESEARCH CENTERS

Medical Research Centres. Harlow, Essex, Longman, biennial.

International Research Centers Directory. Detroit, Gale Research Co., annual.

Research Centers Directory. Detroit, Gale Research Co., annual (updated by *New Research Centers*).

12. SPECIAL LIBRARY COLLECTIONS

Ash, L., comp. *Subject Collections.* 6th ed. New York, R. R. Bowker Co., 1985.

Directory of Special Libraries and Information Centers. Detroit, Gale Research Co., annual (updated by *New Special Libraries*).

PUBLIC POLICY STATEMENT ON THE USE OF ALCOHOL AND OTHER DRUGS DURING PREGNANCY

Background of the Problem

The human fetus is entirely dependent on the maternal environment for its safety, health, growth, and development. Alcohol and other drugs ingested by a pregnant woman may damage the developing fetus by a variety of mechanisms:

1. Alcohol and other drugs cross the placenta and enter the fetal bloodstream, interfering with growth and development both physical and mental, causing reduced birth weight, birth defects, learning and behavior disorders, and newborn distress. The developing fetus cannot detoxify these drugs because of immature enzyme systems.
2. Alcohol and other drugs may interfere with the normal physiological processes of pregnancy, causing fetal loss, prematurity, and obstetrical complications threatening to both maternal and infant health.
3. Acute intoxication due to alcohol or other drug use during pregnancy is associated with motor vehicle accidents, falls, or other trauma to mother and fetus.
4. Alcoholism and other drug dependence during pregnancy, by interfering with nutrition and other health-related behaviors, increase the risks to fetal and maternal health.
5. Physical dependence on alcohol or other drugs at the time of delivery may lead to an alcohol or drug withdrawal syndrome in the newborn infant, as well as to a postpartum withdrawal syndrome in the mother.

6. Alcoholism and other drug dependence in pregnancy, by interfering with interpersonal, occupational, and social functioning, damage the adequacy of the family unit to nurture the resulting infant. Child neglect or abuse may accompany family dysfunction. Alcoholism and other drug dependence may interfere with parent-infant bonding.

Policy Recommendations

In order to prevent harm to mothers and infants, ASAM recommends the following:

1. Widespread and continuing programs to educate the public about the effects of alcohol and other drugs, including tobacco, in pregnancy. These programs should include:

    a. Warning labels in prominent places on alcoholic beverages, nicotine-containing products, over-the-counter drugs, and prescription medicines.
    b. Warning posters at point of sale of alcoholic beverages, nicotine-containing products, and medicines.
    c. Age-appropriate education in elementary and secondary schools, colleges, graduate and professional schools, based on the best available scientific knowledge.
    d. Patient and family education in primary care settings, obstetric-gynecological practices, and in alcoholism and other drug dependency treatment programs.
    e. Public education through community councils on alcoholism and drug dependency and other agencies.

2. Educational materials recommending abstinence from alcohol, for pregnant women, women planning pregnancy and nursing mothers.

3. Improved professional education aimed at early diagnosis of alcoholism and other drug dependence in women in health care settings; and appropriate treatment and referral, including treatment for nicotine dependence.

4. Improved screening for alcoholism and other drug dependence in obstetric practice.
5. The development of close working relationships between obstetric practices, and alcoholism and other drug dependence treatment services, including services for nicotine dependence.
6. Education for obstetricians, pediatricians, family practitioners, and other health professionals, in the management of alcohol and other drug dependent women during pregnancy and delivery, and in the care of infants born to such women, including management of the neonatal withdrawal syndrome.
7. Increased public and private support for research into the effects of alcohol and other drugs on pregnancy and fetal development.

Adopted by ASAM Board of Directors 11/6/88

PUBLIC POLICY STATEMENT ON CHEMICALLY DEPENDENT WOMEN AND PREGNANCY

Background

Because of the adverse effects on fetal development of alcohol and certain other drugs (including nicotine, cocaine, marijuana, and opiates) the chemically dependent woman who is pregnant or may become pregnant is an especially important candidate for intervention and treatment. Similarly, prevention programs should target all women of childbearing age.

Recently, public concern for preventing fetal harm has resulted in punitive measures against pregnant women or women in the postpartum period. These measures have included incarcerating pregnant women in jails to keep them abstinent and the criminal prosecution of mothers for taking drugs while pregnant and thereby passing these substances to the fetus or newborn through the placenta.

The American Society of Addiction Medicine is deeply committed to the prevention of alcohol and other drug-related harm to the health and well-being of children. The most humane and effective way to achieve this end is through education, intervention, and treatment. The imposition of criminal penalties solely because a person suffers from an illness is inappropriate and counterproductive. Criminal prosecution of chemically dependent women will have the overall result of deterring such women from seeking both prenatal care and chemical dependency treatment, thereby increasing, rather than preventing, harm to children and to society as a whole.

Policy Recommendations

The American Society of Addition Medicine supports the following policies:

1. Prevention programs to educate all members of the public about the dangers of alcohol and other drug use during pregnancy and lactation. These should include:

    - Age appropriate school-based education throughout the school curriculum.
    - Public education about alcohol and other drug use in pregnancy and lactation, including health warning labels and posters as well as radio and television messages, educational programs and written materials.
    - Prenatal education about alcohol and other drugs for all pregnant women and significant others, as part of adequate prenatal care.
    - Professional education for all health care professionals, including education of obstetricians and pediatricians in the care of chemically dependent women and their offspring.

2. Early intervention, consultation, and case finding programs specifically designed to reach chemically dependent women:

- Screening for alcohol and other drug problems in all obstetric care services, as well as in all medical settings.
- Adequate case finding, intervention, and referral services for women identified as suffering from chemical dependency.

3. Treatment services able to meet the needs of chemically dependent women:

- Appropriate and accessible chemical dependency treatment services for pregnant women and women of childbearing age and their families, including inpatient and residential treatment. Services to care for the children and newborns of these patients should be provided. Without adequate child care arrangements, chemically dependent women are often unable to engage in the treatment they need.
- Adequate facilities for the outpatient and aftercare phases of treatment for chemically dependent women.
- Adequate perinatal care for chemically dependent women in treatment, sensitive to their special needs.
- Adequate child protection services to provide alternative placement for infants or children of persons suffering from chemical dependency who are unable to function as parents, in the absence of others able to fulfill the parent role.

4. Research:

- Basic and clinical research on the effects of alcohol and other drugs used during pregnancy.
- Model programs, with evaluation component, for case finding intervention and treatment of chemically dependent pregnant women, and for case finding, intervention, and treatment of infants and children affected by maternal alcohol and/or other drug use.

5. Law enforcement:

   - State and local governments should avoid any measures defining alcohol or other drug use during pregnancy as "prenatal child abuse," and should avoid prosecution, jail, or other punitive measures as a substitute for providing effective health services for these women.

6. Preservation of patient confidentiality:

   - No law or regulation should require physicians to violate confidentiality by reporting their pregnant patients to state or local authorities for "prenatal child abuse."

Adopted by ASAM Board of Directors 9/25/89